Michael Torzewski, Karl J. Lackner, Jürgen Bohl, Clemens Sommer

Integrated Cytology of Cerebrospinal Fluid

Michael Torzewski, Karl J. Lackner,
Jürgen Bohl, Clemens Sommer

Integrated Cytology of Cerebrospinal Fluid

With 138 Figures

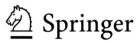 Springer

Michael Torzewski, MD
Institute of Clinical Chemistry and
Laboratory Medicine and Department
of Neuropathology
University of Mainz
55101 Mainz
Germany
torzewski@zentrallabor.klinik.uni-mainz.de

Karl J. Lackner, MD
Institute of Clinical Chemistry
and Laboratory Medicine
University of Mainz
55101 Mainz
Germany
lackner@zentrallabor.klinik.uni-mainz.de

Jürgen Bohl, MD
Department of Neuropathology
University of Mainz
55101 Mainz
Germany
bohl@neuropatho.klinik.uni-mainz.de

Clemens Sommer, MD
Department of Neuropathology
University of Mainz
55101 Mainz
Germany
sommer@neuropatho.klinik.uni-mainz.de

ISBN   978-3-540-75884-6

e-ISBN 978-3-540-75885-3

DOI 10.1007/978-3-540-75885-3

Library of Congress Control Number: 2007938083

© 2008 Springer-Verlag Berlin Heidelberg

springer.com

Springer-Verlag is a part of Springer Science+Business Media

The use of general descriptive names, registered names, trademarks, etc. in this publication does not imply, even in the absence of a specific statement, that such names are exempt from the relevant protective laws and regulations and therefore free for general use.

Product liability: the publishers cannot guarantee the accuracy of any information about dosage and application contained in this book. In every individual case the user must check such information by consulting the relevant literature.

Cover design: Frido Steinen-Broo, eStudio Calamar, Spain

Printed on acid-free paper

5 4 3 2 1 0

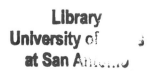

Preface

Cytologic examination of the cerebrospinal fluid (CSF) is a technically simple but productive diagnostic procedure. Its proper performance demands considerable expertise, but it can nevertheless be accomplished relatively rapidly and inexpensively. Therefore, it may be helpful for physicians and also technicians to obtain images of routinely prepared CSF slides of different pathologies. This book will be dedicated to physicians and technicians (both beginners and advanced) who deal with CSF cytology and will assist them with the diagnosis of different pathologies. The term "integrated" of the title implies that we have used immunocytochemical, histological, and immunohistochemical illustrations, gross nervous system pathology, and/or quantitative data liberally in addition to photographs and descriptions of cytologic preparations. This should provide the reader with background knowledge to the significance of abnormal cytological findings in relation to the etiology and pathogenesis of the underlying disease and create a comprehensive picture of the cytopathology of the central nervous system. In particular, we have used several images of immunocytochemical (and also immunohistochemical) illustrations throughout the section "Neoplastic Disorders" (Sect. 6) and suggest useful antibodies for further immunocytological work-up in cases where the routine cytological examination of CSF alone does not yield a sufficiently precise cytological diagnosis. This emphasis mirrors the widespread application of immunocytochemistry to CSF in the diagnosis of neoplastic diseases.

The book is systematically organized according to diagnostic categories, i.e., common cell types, inflammatory conditions, non-neoplastic disorders, neoplastic disorders, and contaminants. We have also provided a brief description of cytologic techniques (CSF cell preparation and common artifacts). However, as a more detailed description is far beyond the scope of the present book, the reader is referred to the appropriate literature. In each chapter, the images are accompanied by a brief introduction and description on the opposing page. If not otherwise specified CSF samples are stained by the panoptic Pappenheim's stain (a combination of the May–Grünwald's eosin-methylene blue stain with the Giemsa azure II-eosin stain) and shown using an oil immersion objective (×100).

Histologic specimens are usually stained with hematoxylin and eosin (H&E) and shown using a × 40 objective.

The authors would be glad to receive suggestions as to how the book might be further improved. In this regard, submissions of additional illustrations or of cytological preparations showing uncommon but diagnostically relevant findings would be particularly helpful. We thank Springer-Verlag GmbH, Heidelberg, Germany, and in particular Ellen Blasig and Gabriele Schröder for their extensive help and advice during the preparation of this book. We are grateful to Andreas Kreft, MD, Institute of Pathology, University of Mainz, for the critical reading of Sect. 6.3. We also thank the technical staff of the Institute of Clinical Chemistry and Laboratory Medicine and the Department of Neuropathology, University of Mainz, for the preparation of the cytological and histologic specimens.

Mainz, Germany   **Michael Torzewski**
August 2007   **Karl J. Lackner**
                                                        Jürgen Bohl
                                                   Clemens Sommer

Contents

CHAPTER 1

Cerebrospinal Fluid Cell Preparation

1.1 General Considerations

Since the cellular component of CSF obtained from the lumbar area is generally scant, an efficient method of concentrating this material is necessary. Furthermore, considerations regarding the selection of cytopreparation techniques include the potential for cell loss, the clarity of cellular detail, and the spectrum of stains offered. The most commonly utilized methods today are membrane filtration and cytocentrifugation.

1

1.2 Cytocentrifugation

Of all the possible methods of transferring cells from CSF samples onto slides, most laboratories now use a cytospin apparatus, such as the Shandon cytocentrifuge (Fig. 1A, reprinted by kind permission of Thermo Shandon), which is efficient in terms of cell yield. The cytocentrifuge technique also allows use of virtually all types of fixation and staining, including the preparation of cells for immunocytochemistry, immunofluorescence and in situ hybridization. Because of the centrifugal force when in the running position, the cytofunnel will raise up in vertical position (right-hand side of the illustration). When the cytospin is not running the cytofunnel is loaded at an angle to prevent the specimen coming into contact with the filter card (left-hand side of the illustration; blue color, specimen). To load the slide clip with a re-useable sample chamber and filter card (Fig. 1B, reprinted by kind permission of Thermo Shandon) it is necessary to fit the glass slide (1), to fit the filter card (2), to fit the re-useable sample chamber (3), and finally to pull up the spring and press it into the two retaining hooks to hold the chamber in place (4). After running the cytospin, cytospin sample chambers are unloaded and samples are fixed as soon as possible to avoid autolysis. The specimen can now be stained and examined microscopically.

A

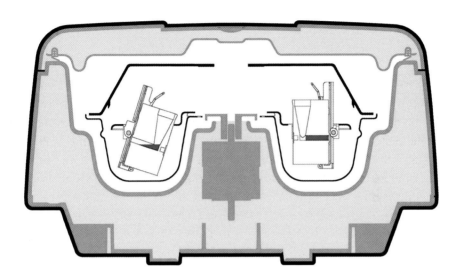

B

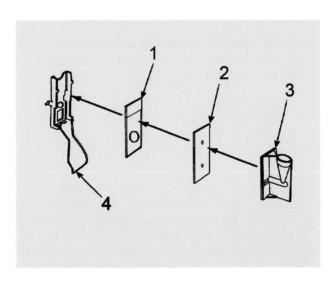

CHAPTER 2

Common Artifacts

2.1 General Considerations

Several preanalytical and analytical pitfalls may cause artifacts, making proper assessment of the CSF cell preparation impossible or at least more difficult. First of all, it is important to ensure that CSF samples reach the laboratory as soon as possible after the puncture (within 2 h). If this is not possible, fixation of the CSF sample with buffered formalin (1:1) is an option, but should not be routinely performed. The storage temperature of native CSF should be between 5°C and 12°C to minimize cell damage. Lower temperatures may lead to cold lysis, whereas higher temperatures accelerate catabolic mechanisms [1].

2

2.2 Autolysis, High Cell Concentration, Unproper Loading, Adhesion

Slide preparation must be quick because cells in CSF deteriorate rapidly. Because of its limited buffering capacity (especially if exposed to air) [1] and its low protein content, the CSF offers an unsuitable medium for living cells. Elevated pH and low oncotic pressure causes some cells to swell, some to perish and others to become unrecognizable (Fig. 2A). Cytology specimens are often submitted to the laboratory with a cell concentration that is too high for cytospin preparations until diluted (Fig. 2B, objective × 40). As a general rule, the concentration chosen should be such that the cells within the sample have adequate space to spread into a monolayer on the slide surface with minimal overlap. These concentrated specimens should therefore first be evaluated for cell number and then be diluted to an approximate cell concentration by the addition of a balanced electrolyte solution. It is important to use a fluid that has a proper osmolarity, in order not to introduce structural changes into the cell sample. Simple solutions of sodium chloride (0.9% saline) are unsuitable as diluents – they produce rapid changes in nuclear chromatin and interfere with subsequent cytological evaluation. If the cytoclip slide clip is not loaded properly (see Sect. 1), i.e., the glass slide oriented with the frosted side to the top and the frosted label end toward the cytofunnel, cells will be deposited not in the defined area, but rather on the other end of the glass slide (Fig. 2C, objective × 2.50).

Due to the methodology of sample preparation (centrifugation) artificial adhesion of cells is a common phenomenon (Fig. 2D) and should not be misinterpreted as clusters of tumor cells or, in the case of a monocyte surrounded by several erythrocytes, as the initial stage of erythrophagocytosis.

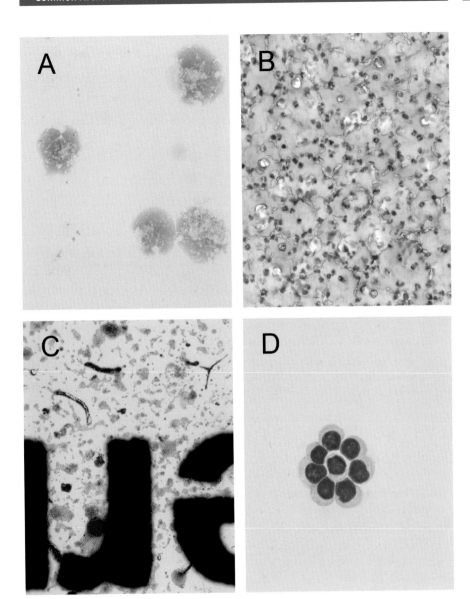

CHAPTER 3

The Common Cell Types of Cerebrospinal Fluid

3.1 General Considerations

The subarachnoid space is a fluid-filled cavity that covers the brain and spinal cord and communicates with the internal ventricles of the brain. It is bound externally by a fine arachnoid membrane and internally by the pial surface of the brain, and normally contains only a loose fibrovascular stroma. The arachnoid membrane and pia mater are the two membranous layers that comprise the leptomeninges. CSF is produced within the ventricular system by cells of the choroid plexus and ependyma [2], and passes out of the ventricular system at the base of the brain into the subarachnoid space by means of the foramina of Luschka and Magendie. A specimen of CSF taken in the lumbar area and unaltered by diseases of the central nervous system normally contains two types of cells, i.e., lymphocytic and monocytic forms. The ratio of lymphocytes to monocytes is about 70 to 30 [3, 4]. Since the puncture needle penetrates the skin, adipose and fibrous tissue, and striated muscle, and since the cartilage and bones of the vertebral column may be also in the path of the needle, non-neoplastic cellular elements, such as squamous cells, adipose and fibrous tissue, and striated muscle, as well as chondrocytes and cells of the hemopoietic system, are sometimes carried in the specimen. A specimen taken from the ventricular area may also contain fragments of cerebral cortex, white matter, and ependymal cells, as the needle traverses all of these structures.

3.2 Lymphocytic Cell Forms

3.2.1 Non-activated Lymphocytic Cell Forms

3

A specimen of CSF taken in the lumbar area and unaltered by diseases of the central nervous system normally contains two types of cells: lymphocytic and monocytic forms. The ratio of lymphocytes to monocytes is about 70 to 30 [3, 4]. Therefore, small numbers of lymphocytes are seen in most CSF samples. These are small (5–8 μm in diameter), relatively isomorphic cells. Usually, the nuclear chromatin is dense and homogeneous (Fig. 3.2A). Occasionally, they show a discrete but ill-defined paler structure within the nucleus, which is the nucleolus (Fig. 3.2B, arrowhead). There is little cytoplasm, which is pale blue and clear (Fig. 3.2A,B, 1), or sometimes slightly more intense (Fig. 3.2B, 2).

Immunophenotyping of lymphocytes by flow cytometry revealed that in normal CSF, CD3$^+$ T lymphocytes constitute the vast majority of CSF lymphocytes (about 93%), while the numbers of B lymphocytes and natural killer (NK) cells are low [5].

3.2.2 Activated Lymphocytic Cell Forms

Activated lymphocytic cell forms are part of the differentiation of normal B lymphocytes from plasma cells under inflammatory conditions. Compared with non-activated lymphocytic cell forms, these are larger (up to 25 μm in diameter) or dark cytoplasmic forms with a more pronounced cytoplasmic border (Fig. 3.2C, 1; D, 1) and/or more lightly stained and somewhat heterogeneous nuclear chromatin (Fig. 3.2C, 2). These cytologic features may sometimes lead to confusion with the malignant hematopoietic cells of lymphoma or leukemia (see Sect. 6.3). Immunophenotyping of these reactive cells is particularly helpful, because mixtures of reactive T and B lymphocytes are inevitably demonstrated, in contrast to the monoclonal population that is present in the case of malignant lymphoma. Plasma cells (Fig. 3.2C, 3) are never present in normal CSF, i.e., their presence always indicates an inflammation of the central nervous system (CNS). The nucleus of mature plasma cells is excentrically located and contains a grainy chromatin structure. A crescent-shaped area of light cytoplasm around the nucleus is typical, but not present in every case. Due to enhanced proliferation, sometimes mitoses (Fig. 3.2D, 2) or binuclear cells can be observed.

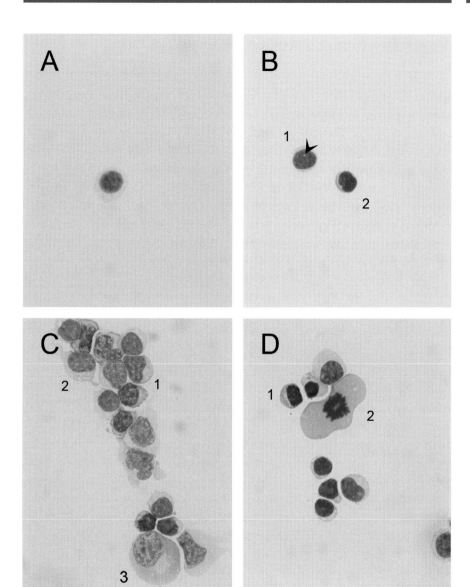

3

3.3 Monocytic Cell Forms

The monocytic cell forms normally degenerate more rapidly in vitro than do the lymphocytic cell forms. Monocytic cell forms have a hematogenic (monocyto-poietic) origin [6]. The cells are large (15–20 μm in diameter) and have an eccentric, oval, kidney-shaped or horseshoe-shaped, blue–gray nucleus, which often contains large, pale nucleoli (Fig. 3.3A,B, arrowhead). The cytoplasm is pale blue–gray, occasionally interspersed with vacuoles. Larger and/or numerous cytoplasmic vacuoles are already a sign of a higher activation state (Fig. 3.3C,D). Furthermore, compared with non-activated monocytic cell forms, activated monocytes are larger and their nucleus sometimes more rounded (Fig. 3.3C, D). Also in Fig. 3.3C, 1 and D, 1, note the presence of erythrocytes.

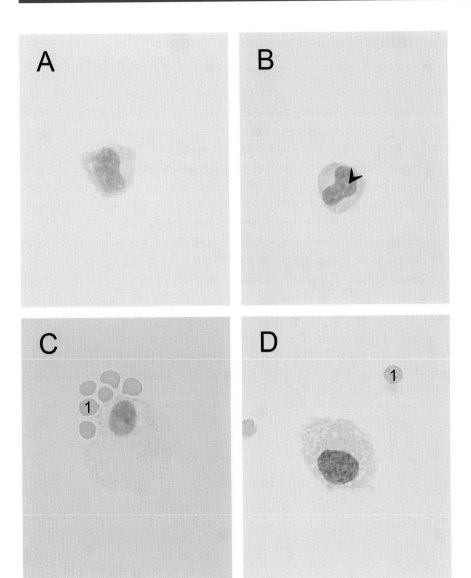

3

3.4 Macrophages

Monocyte-derived macrophages survive days or even months and are indicative of a pathologic process; hence their diagnostic value. Their primary function is the elimination of foreign matter by means of phagocytosis. These foreign elements may be of various sizes and either living (cells [Fig. 3.4A: intact erythrocytes and erythrocytes that have lost their characteristic color and appear as empty vacuoles due to the enzymatic digestion of hemoglobin], bacteria [Fig. 3.4D, arrowhead: staphylococci], viruses) or non-living (pigments [Fig. 3.4B, arrowhead: hemosiderin, Fig. 3.4C: hematoidin, arrow], lipids, and substances given intrathecally). According to the ingested material, one can distinguish among erythrophages (Fig. 3.4A), siderophages (Fig. 3.4B), bacteriophages (Fig. 3.4D), leukophages, lipophages, etc. The cells usually appear singly, but can be found in rather large groups (Fig. 3.4C). The nucleus can be either centrally or excentrically located, and one or more nucleoli are often present (Fig. 3.4C, arrowheads). Deposits of various sorts of phagocytized material can often be found in the cytoplasm (Fig. 3.4C, arrow: hematoidin). The life span of the phagocytes is relatively long, e.g., siderophages (Fig. 3.4B) can persist in the subarachnoid space up to 120 days after the initial hemorrhage in some cases [7].

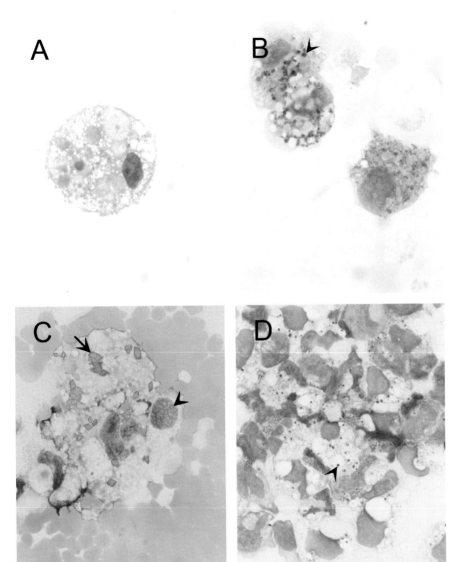

3

3.5 Plexus Epithelial and Ependymal Cells

Cells from the choroid plexus (Fig. 3.5B: histologic specimen) and the cuboidal or columnar ependymal cells that line the ventricles (Fig. 3.5D: histologic specimen, oil immersion) are normal brain elements that have ready access to CSF. They occasionally occur singularly or in papillary clusters in CSF obtained by lumbar puncture from normal individuals. Cytologic differentiation between cells of the ependyma and those of the choroid plexus is hardly possible. Plexus epithelial cells usually appear as clusters of several cells with wide, coarse-grained cytoplasm and uniform, round to slightly oval nuclei (Fig. 3.5A). Ependymal cells are rather fragile cells with round, often pyknotic-appearing nuclei and a wide border of pink or blue–gray cytoplasm, occasionally interspersed with vacuoles (Fig. 3.5C, surrounded by many erythrocytes). Both cell types appear more frequently in the CSF of small children and in cases of hydrocephalus, as well as in samples obtained by ventricular puncture. Ependymal and choroidal cells also appear in the CSF sample after intrathecal administration of drugs, especially of cytostatics. They are generally of little diagnostic value. However, these cells may be morphologically changed in reaction to an appropriate stimulus, and may therefore be a source of error in diagnostic material.

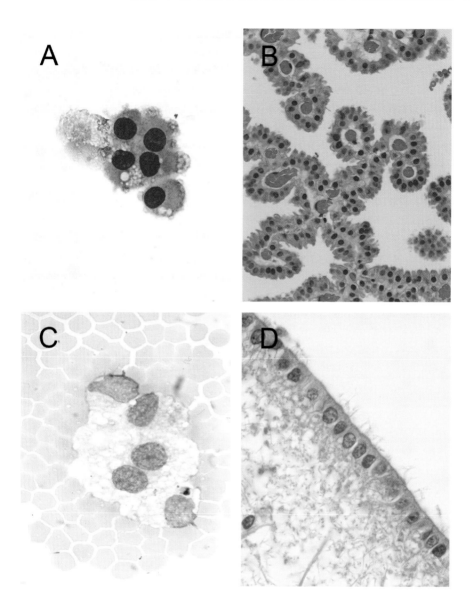

3.6 Arachnoidal Cells

The subarachnoid space (Fig. 3.6A: histologic specimen, SAS) is lined externally by the arachnoid membrane, which is composed of meningothelial cells (Fig. 3.6A, arrowhead). The arachnoid membrane of normal individuals sometimes contains focal proliferations of these cells, which are termed meningothelial rests. Groups of meningothelial cells also comprise the tips of the arachnoid granulations, which are protrusions from the SAS into the dural sinuses. Arachnoidal cells are occasionally seen in CSF from normal individuals (Fig. 3.6B,C), and they are probably derived from either meningothelial rests or arachnoid granulations. The cells usually show a wide, pink or violet, sometimes reticular cytoplasm and uniform, more or less oval nuclei. Rarely, they are seen in moderate numbers, raising the possibility of a meningioma (Fig. 3.6D: histologic specimen of a meningothelial meningioma, WHO grade I). However, the presence of arachnoidal cells in CSF is not in itself diagnostic of meningioma in the absence of a clinically detectable mass.

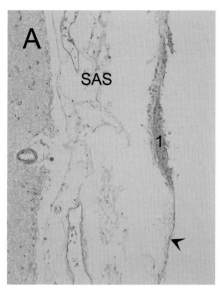

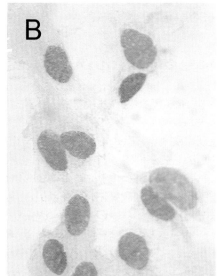

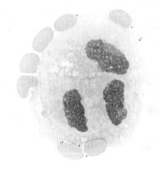

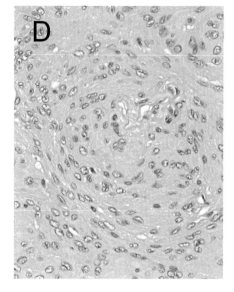

3.7 Accidental Findings

3.7.1 Chondrocytes

Cells that originate in the path of the aspiration needle are sometimes found in a specimen. A frequent finding of lumbar puncture-derived CSF is the chondrocyte. These cells enter the CSF as a result of an injury to the cartilage of a vertebra caused by the puncture needle. Usually, they show a typical appearance with an intensely red cytoplasm and uniform, round to slightly oval nuclei (Fig. 3.7.1A). Since these cells originate from bradytrophic tissue, they are rather stable, even if all other cell types are already autolytic due to inappropriate processing of the sample. In CSF cell preparations obtained from patients with degenerative changes of the cartilage (Fig. 3.7.1D: histologic specimen with chondrocyte "cloning" (1) and granular change as evidence of degeneration and/or prolapse, objective × 20), they sometimes appear in clusters (Fig. 3.7.1B) or even may be mistaken for neoplastic cells (Fig. 3.7.1C). The presence of these cells in CSF, however, has no known pathologic significance.

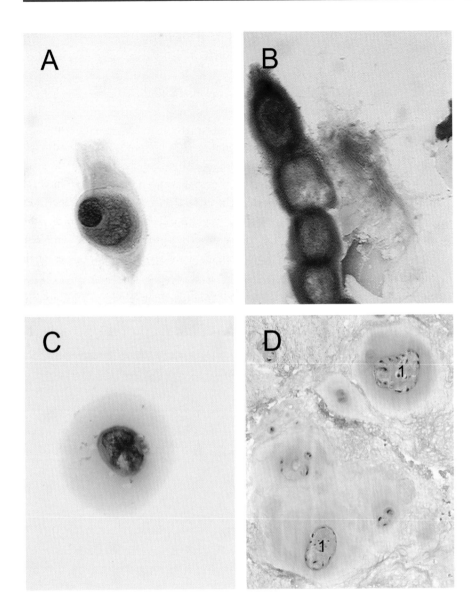

3

3.7.2 Squamous Epithelial Cells, Artificial Bleeding, and Cells of the Hemopoietic System

Non-neoplastic cellular elements, such as squamous epithelial cells (Fig. 3.7.2A, sometimes in rather large groups and with bacterial contamination), presumably from the skin (Fig. 3.7.2B: histologic specimen), may occasionally be found. Sometimes, even fragments of capillaries, striated muscle, and adipose and fibrous tissue are carried in from subcutaneous tissue or muscle.

Artificial blood contamination (Fig. 3.7.2C) may be difficult to distinguish from subarachnoid hemorrhage (see Sect. 5.3). However, it is easily recognizable immediately after puncture (three-glass test) and the erythrocyte/leukocyte ratio is similar to that of peripheral blood.

Sometimes, immature cells of the hematopoietic system are found in the CSF of small children and cachectic, elderly patients, even if leukemia is not present (Fig. 3.7.2D: 1, proerythroblast; 2, eosinophilic metamyelocyte; 3, basophilic erythroblast; 4, polychromatic erythroblast). These cells enter the CSF as a result of an injury to the marrow of a vertebra caused by the puncture needle. This may cause initial confusion, but the simultaneous presence of cells of the myelopoietic, erythropoietic, and/or thrombopoietic systems usually indicates the source of this condition.

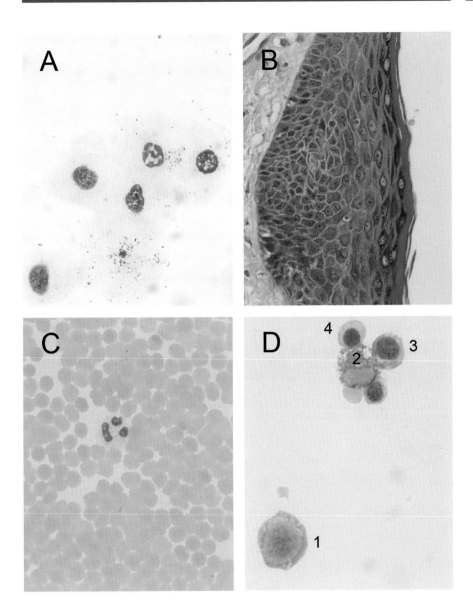

CHAPTER 4

Inflammatory Conditions

4.1 General Considerations

Inflammatory disorders, especially infections of the CNS usually induce severe changes in the cellular content of the CSF. Nearly all types of infection may involve the CNS: bacterial, viral, and mycotic infections (fungi), diseases of the CNS caused by protozoa, and even metazoal parasitic invasions of the brain and its coverings, which are not uncommon in some tropical regions. Additionally, several autoimmunological diseases may lead to a cellular response in the CSF.

As a rule, acute bacterial, fungal, and also protozoal infections induce mainly a polymorphonuclear leukocytic response in the cellular content of the CSF, but this may be misleading in otherwise necrotizing cerebral processes (e.g., in peracute viral infections). Later on these infections also show lymphocytes, activated monocytes, and macrophages. Acute tuberculous meningitis may also be characterized by polymorphonuclear granulocytes; in later stages lymphocytic cell forms will prevail.

On the other hand, a cytopathological picture predominantly showing lymphocytic cells and also plasma cells hints at a viral infection (or a borreliosis). In former times, abundant plasma cells in the CSF were suspected to indicate a syphilitic infection; nowadays this is a rare event.

These observations are only faint indications as to the special type of underlying infection. In all cases it should be attempted to identify the infectious agent by culture, by measuring the antibody titers and/or by polymerase chain reaction (PCR).

The cellular pattern of the CSF alterations changes rapidly according to the definite stage of the infection, and it also reflects the success of specific or unspecific therapy. A large amount of eosinophilic granulocytes is a hint at a parasitic infection, such as cysticercosis. Some viral infections lead to a higher content of

4

atypical lymphoid or lymphoblastic cells in the CSF, perhaps making the differential diagnosis from a neoplastic process of the lymphatic system very difficult.

Intracellular inclusions, characteristic of a viral infection, are only rarely found in the CSF. Definite identification of an infectious disease of the CNS must take into consideration the results of all the different methods of clinical and laboratory diagnostics.

4.2 Bacterial Infections

Many different bacteria are able to induce severe acute or subacute leptomeningitis. Among the microorganisms that cause purulent phlegmonous inflammation of the arachnoid are meningococci, streptococci, *Haemophilus influenzae* type b, and others.

The laboratory investigation of the CSF reveals heavily increased cell numbers (usually >1,000 leukocytes/µl). At the beginning, most of the inflammatory cells are neutrophilic leukocytes. Very often they contain many microorganisms in their cytoplasm.

Figure 4.2A shows typical diplococci in the leukocytic cytoplasm (arrowheads; 1, activated lymphocyte), sometimes even small packages of four bacteria; the meningitis was caused by *Neisseria meningitidis*. In the later stages of bacterial leptomeningitis the cellular population exhibits more and more activated monocytes and macrophages, as shown in Fig. 4.2B and C. Figure 4.2B shows a macrophage (1) containing coagulase-negative staphylococci (arrowheads). In Fig. 4.2C, large amounts of small lanceolate diplococci can be seen, sometimes surrounded by a small unstained halo, corresponding to a capsule (arrowheads). These are typical signs of a pneumococcal infection, caused by *Streptococcus pneumoniae*. These bacteria prove to be Gram-positive (stained dark blue) after Gram staining (Fig. 4.2D).

Exact identification of bacteria is only possible by microbiological investigation, which should include determination of resistance.

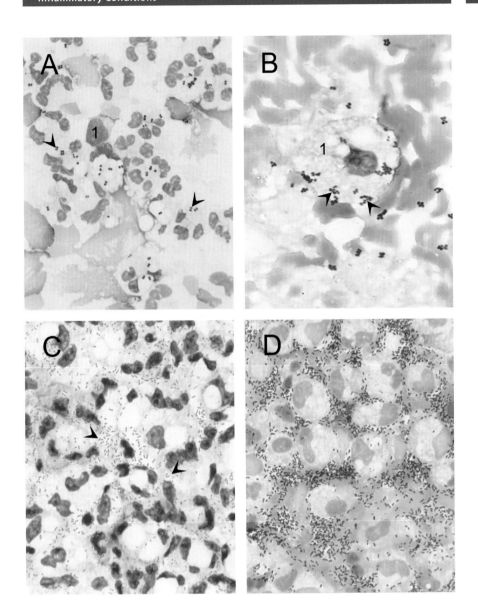

4

4.3   Viral Infections

4.3.1   Viral Meningitis and Meningoencephalitis

Acute viral infections of the CNS usually involve both the central nervous tissue and the leptomeninges, e.g., infections with the herpes simplex virus, Coxsackie virus or influenza virus.

At the beginning of the necrotizing process in the cerebral cortical areas and/or in the brainstem nuclei there might be on the first day mainly polymorphonuclear leukocytes in the CSF as a consequence of a severe necrotizing damage of the brain tissue. After that, lymphocytic cells will predominate in the CSF (Fig. 4.3.1A,B). In addition to normal lymphocytes (Fig. 4.3.1A, 1), there are activated cells (Fig. 4.3.1A, 2), lymphoblastic elements (Fig. 4.3.1A, 3), and sometimes even some mitoses. Later on, the cytopathologic picture additionally shows plasma cells (B, 1), activated monocytes (B, 2), and macrophages.

Figure 4.3.1C shows the macroscopic appearance of acute severe herpes simplex encephalitis with hemorrhagic necrotizing alterations, mainly in the temporal lobe. The damage is not always totally symmetrical; in this case, the left side is more severely involved.

In the brain tissue the inflammatory infiltrations are found around small blood vessels and cuffing the capillaries and small veins (Fig. 4.3.1D, objective ×10). As there is continuity between the perivascular Virchow–Robin spaces and the subarachnoid compartment of the CSF, the inflammatory cells can easily move from inside the brain tissue into the surrounding leptomeninges and, furthermore, into the spinal channel.

Very often, acute generalized viral infections of the whole organism are accompanied by slight concomitant leptomeningitis with disseminated lymphocytic infiltrations in the subarachnoid space and also in the Virchow–Robin spaces of the cerebral parenchyma.

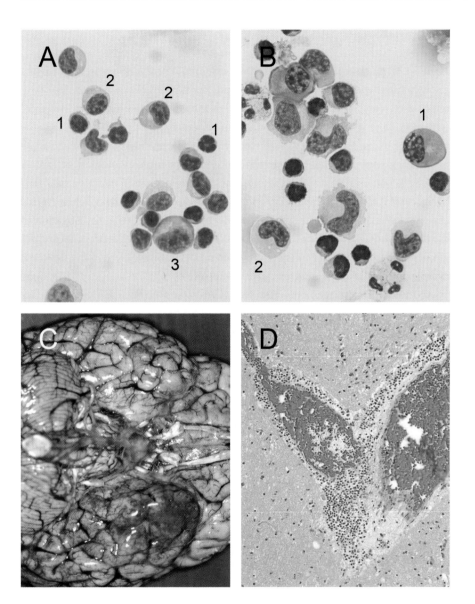

4

4.3.2 Rabies

Figure 4.3.2A (objective × 20) shows the cytopathological findings in the CSF of a young patient with an acute rabies virus infection. As CSF was obtained very early after onset, the CSF still shows typical alterations of an acute bacterial infection, with more than 700 cells/µl. There were mainly neutrophilic granulocytes (1), some macrophages, and only a few activated lymphocytic elements. Obviously, acute necrotizing viral encephalitis sometimes presents the same cytologic reactions in the CSF as bacterial meningitis. The correct diagnosis of a viral infection may only be successful by directly demonstrating the viral antigen in macrophages. In this case, the final diagnosis of rabies was found by the post-mortem investigation of the brain. There were typical Negri bodies (Fig. 4.3.2B, arrowheads) in several regions of the isocortex and in some brain stem nuclei, shown here in the neuronal cytoplasm in cells of the nucleus olivaris inferior.

Abundant viral antigen could be detected with a specific antibody against rabies. Figure 4.3.2C shows a midbrain region with severe involvement of perikarya, nerve cell processes, and to a lower degree, of astrocytes and activated microglia. Negri bodies also seem to give a positive reaction (arrowhead).

The detection of viral antigen by means of an immunofluorescence procedure proved to be even more sensitive (Fig. 4.3.2D), with a positive reaction in nearly all types of neurons in an isocortical area.

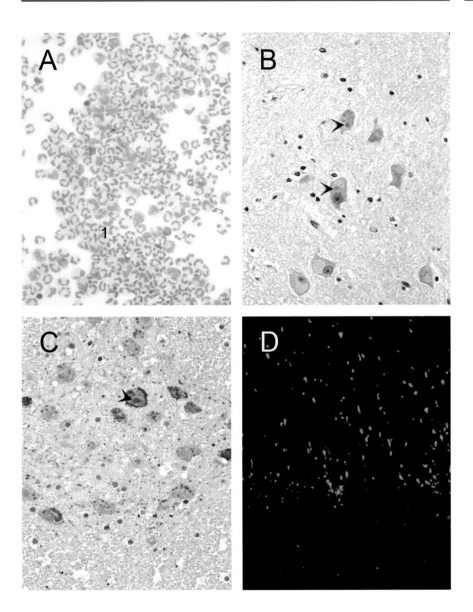

4.4 Fungal Infections

Fungal infections are also a very common additional finding in immunosuppressed or immunodeficient patients. Furthermore, they have been found to be an undesired side effect of prolonged antibiotic therapy.

In yeast infections, the single fungal bodies are floating freely in the CSF and can be detected by investigating the usual cytologic specimen.

In Fig. 4.4.1A, a single yeast body is surrounded by a broad mucous capsule (1). In the neighborhood there are many neutrophilic granulocytes (2) and some activated lymphoid cells (3). Staining with periodic acid (PAS; Fig. 4.4.1B) illustrates typical budding of yeast cell bodies (arrowhead).

The mycotic infection mainly spreads along the pathway of the CSF. In Fig. 4.4.1C and D, histologic specimens of the brain are shown, stained using Grocott's methenamine silver. In Fig. 4.4.1C (objective ×10), the meshwork of the subarachnoid space is filled with fungi and they spread along the perivascular Virchow–Robin spaces into the brain parenchyma. There is also – in this case – no inflammatory reaction as a consequence of the immunodeficient state of the patient (congenital immunodeficiency). At a higher magnification (Fig. 4.4.1D), abundant fungal bodies, stained black, fill the spaces between the network of the arachnoid tissue. Typical budding is found in many areas (arrowhead).

In contrast to yeast infections, mold fungal infections are not very often found in the cytologic specimens of the CSF, because the extending hyphal structures are in most cases more intensely fixed to histologic structures such as blood vessels, collagen-containing fibrous tissue, and also cerebral or spinal tissue. The formation of spores in the central nervous system is not possible; this can only happen in the presence of oxygen-containing air, e.g., in the nasal or sinusoidal cavities and in the lungs. The most common species found in mold fungal infections in man belong to the *Aspergillus* group; however, recently, infections with mucorales seem to have become more common than before.

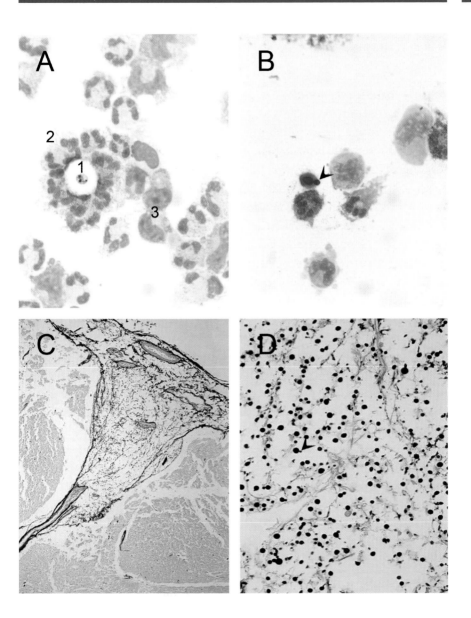

4.5 Parasites

4.5.1 *Toxoplasma gondii*

The activation of a latent infection with the protozoon *Toxoplasma gondii* (the term "gondii" seems to be inappropriate; the germ was first found in small laboratory animals in the north of Africa, in a rodent named "gundi" and not "gondi") is a very common finding in immunosuppressed patients with severe malignancies or in patients with HIV infections.

Figure 4.5.1A shows several tachyzoites of *Toxoplasma gondii*. Surrounded by erythrocytes (1), supposedly artificial contamination, the protozoal microorganisms (2) fill the cytoplasm of a phagocytic cell (3) and float freely in the CSF as well (2). In Fig. 4.5.1B, the infectious agents are stained with a specific polyclonal antibody. They are found as single tiny organisms (1) or as a pseudocystic accumulation of tachyzoites (2).

These characteristic pseudocystic toxoplasmic bodies can also be found in histologic specimens in many regions of the central nervous system (Fig. 4.5.1C, 1); they represent resting forms of the infectious agent and may release the tachyzoites during an acute reactivation of the disease. In areas of necrotizing encephalitic alterations the tissue contains many toxoplasmic protozoa, detected by immunohistochemistry (Fig. 4.5.1D, arrowheads, objective × 10). There is nearly no inflammatory reaction as a consequence of the underlying immunosuppressed or immunodeficient state of the patient.

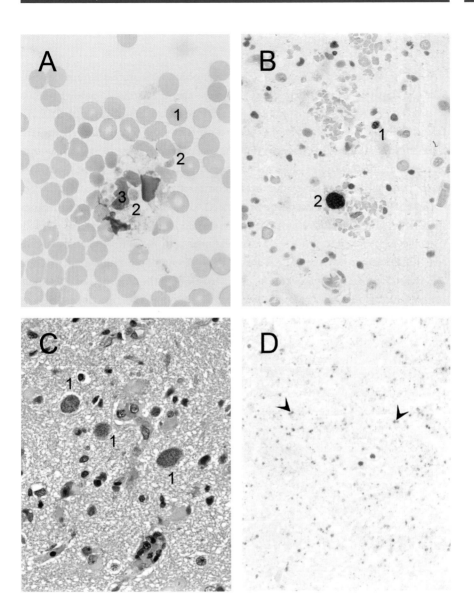

4.5.2   Acanthamoeba

Free-living amoebae (FLA) of the genus Acanthamoeba are distributed world-wide and have been described as the causative agents of granulomatous amebic encephalitis (GAE), amebic keratitis, and skin infections. Most cases of GAE reported in the literature were diagnosed postmortem. Even with various treatment regimens, the outcome has been fatal in the majority of reports.

In routine CSF cytology (Fig. 4.5.2A, objective × 20, B) amoebic trophozoites are characterized by a small nucleus with prominent central nucleolus (Fig. 4.5.2B, arrowhead) and digestive vacuoles (Fig. 4.5.2B, arrow), some of which may sometimes be filled with bacteria (not shown). It should be noted that the cells vaguely resemble macrophages and may be misclassified. In an aliquot of native CSF (Fig. 4.5.2C) trophozoites can be detected by differential interference microscopy (arrowhead: contractile vacuole). In order to confirm the presence of FLA, cultures should be initiated on various media that support the growth of different genera of FLA. The organism shown here was classified as group II Acanthamoeba on the basis of the cyst morphology (Fig. 4.5.2D, objective ×20). Sequence analysis of the 18S rRNA gene showed closest homology to the Acanthamoeba sequence group T4 [8].

Figure 4.5.2 is reprinted by kind permission of the *Journal of Clinical Microbiology.*

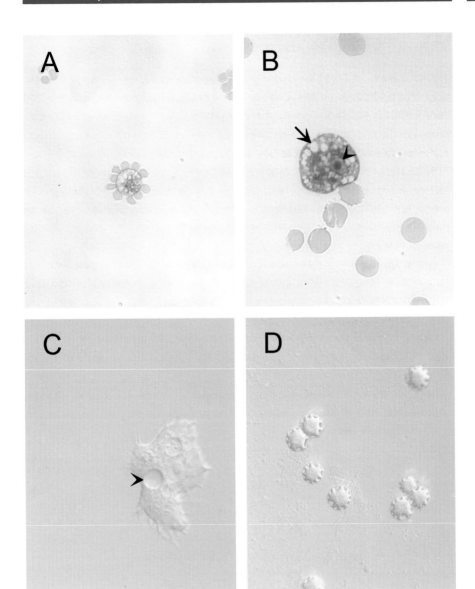

4.5.3   Leishmaniasis

Diseases caused by protozoa are very common all over the world, e.g., American and African trypanosomiasis, cutaneous and visceral leishmaniasis, malaria and toxoplasmosis, and furthermore pneumocystosis, babesiosis, amebiasis, balantidiasis, giardiasis, coccidiosis, and microsporidiosis.

It is surely a rare event that protozoa are found in the CSF obtained by lumbar puncture; but sometimes they can be found in a sanguinolent sample of the CSF. Figure 4.5.3A–D shows a specimen of a patient with Leishmaniasis (visceral form: Kala-Azar, which is Hindi and means "black fever"). While entering the human body the organisms in their promastigote form usually turn over into the smaller amastigote type.

Figure 4.5.3A shows many intracellular (1) and also some extracellular (2) leishmaniasis. The organisms appear larger in cytologic specimens than in tissue specimens. Nuclei and kinetoplasts are distinct in these forms of leishmaniasis. There is also one promastigote organism (3).

Figure 4.5.3B–D shows single forms of extracellular leishmaniasis (Fig. 4.5.3B, 1) amidst damaged erythrocytes (Fig. 4.5.3C, 1) and single lymphocytes (Fig. 4.5.3B, 2; D, 1).

As a consequence of the increase in world-wide travel and climate change, a higher frequency of tropical diseases will be probably be observed in the future, even in temperate zones.

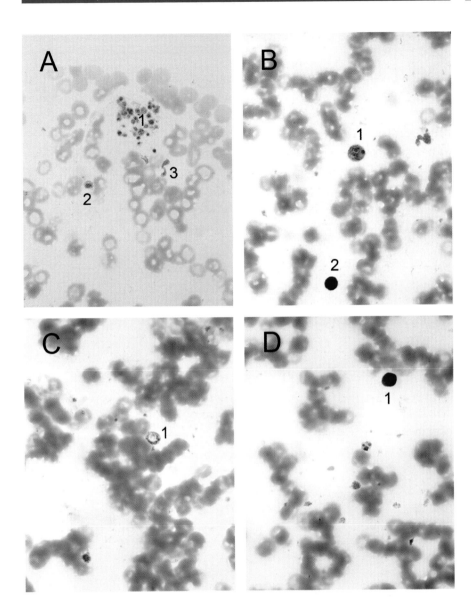

CHAPTER 5

Non-neoplastic Disorders

5.1 General Considerations

Non-neoplastic disorders of the CNS cover a wide range of different entities. These include vascular disorders such as cerebral infarction and hemorrhage, as well as the large group of demyelinating disorders. Many of them show only a few if any cytologic CSF abnormalities, especially in cases of slow chronic processes. With the exception of hemorrhage, the cellular changes are usually rather nonspecific, so that the diagnosis does not depend on CSF cytology. However, cytology may support the suspected diagnosis. Cells present in the CSF of patients with non-neoplastic disorders are monocytes with signs of activation or macrophages with phagocytosed material. If inflammation is present, there may be activated lymphocytes or plasma cells, as in multiple sclerosis. Granulocytes are absolutely uncommon in these disorders and should alert the cytologist to other potential diagnoses, especially infectious disorders.

5

5.2 Infarction

Cerebral infarction is accompanied by nonspecific changes in CSF composition and cytology. Activated monocytes with signs of phagocytosis are present in many cases (Fig. 5.2A). However, in contrast to hemorrhage, the phagocytic vacuoles are small and the origin of the phagocytosed material cannot be identified. Cell number is usually low (<20 μl) if the infarct is purely ischemic. The presence of numerous granulocytes should alert the cytologist to the possibility of bacterial embolism, e.g., in the course of endocarditis. Beginning on the second day after infarction, there may be mild to moderate impairment of the blood–CSF barrier with increased CSF–serum ratios of albumin (Fig. 5.2B). Figure 5.2C represents an H&E stain of an infarct showing numerous monocytes/macrophages in the infarct zone (1). Immunohistochemical staining for neurofilament (Fig. 5.2D) shows complete loss of neurons in the infarcted area (1) with practically no residual staining. This is quite different from acute demyelinating disease, where mainly myelin sheaths are phagocytosed (see Sect. 5.4.2). The activated monocytes in CSF are supposed to originate from the cell population in the infarcted area.

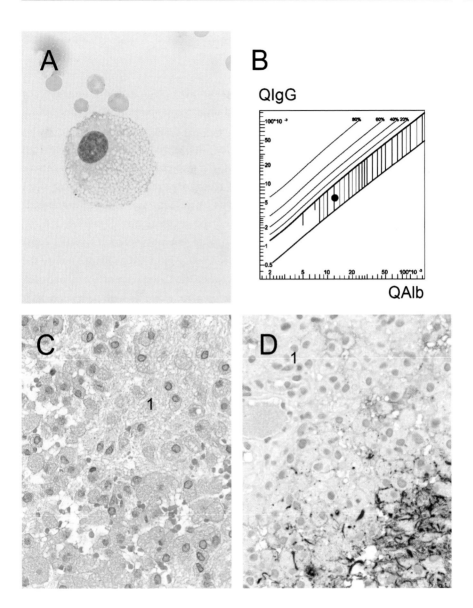

5

5.3 Hemorrhage

An extraordinary leptomeningeal cell reaction takes place if blood infiltrates the CSF, as may result from trauma, ruptured aneurysm, spontaneous intracerebral hemorrhage (hypertension or coagulopathy), hemorrhagic infarct, arteriovenous malformation, tumor or other rare diseases. The presence of blood as a foreign material causes aseptic/chemical meningitis. In rare cases, the pleocytosis can attain levels of 1,500 cells/µl, the majority of which are granulocytes. The first signs of phagocytosis appear about 2–3 h after the introduction of blood into the CSF. Degradation of the hemoglobin begins, and the erythrocytes (Fig. 5.3A, 1; C, 1; D, 1) lose their characteristic color and appear as empty vacuoles in the cytoplasm of the macrophages (Fig. 5.3A, arrowhead). About 4 days elapse before the appearance of the first hemosiderin granules in the cytoplasm of the phagocyte. The digested hemoglobin is stored in the cytoplasm, either as hemosiderin, which contains iron, or as iron-free hematoidin. The hemosiderin appears in the cytoplasm in the form of dark brown to gray–black or blue granules, which are sometimes quite large (Fig. 5.3B, arrowheads). However, as in melanoma metastases of the CNS, the phagocytes are capable of depositing both hemosiderin and melanin in the cytoplasm; staining with Prussian blue provides the only definite evidence of hemosiderin in the cytoplasm (Fig. 5.3C). Iron-free hematoidin (bilirubin), the final stage of hemoglobin breakdown, is deposited in the cytoplasm after 8 days, usually as brownish yellow crystals (Fig. 5.3D, arrowheads). Isolated crystals of hematoidin can sometimes be found in the CSF when the macrophages degenerate. The life span of the phagocytes is relatively long, and they can persist in the subarachnoid space for up to 120 days after the initial hemorrhage [7].

In addition to providing evidence of a single hemorrhage, even several months after the event, macrophages can also indicate repeated hemorrhage. In this case, recently ingested erythrocytes, bleached erythrocytes, hemosiderin, and hematoidin are simultaneously present in the cytoplasm.

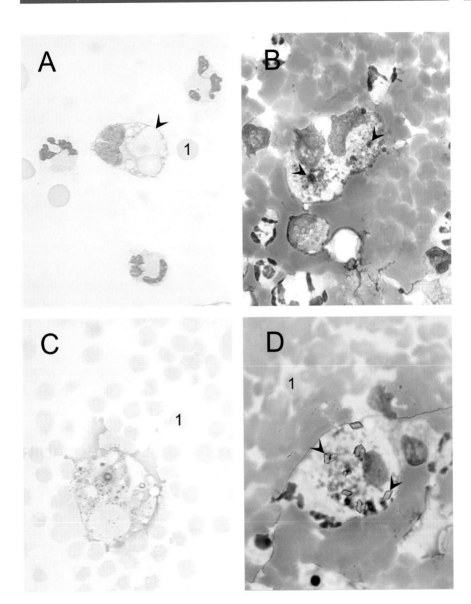

5.4 Demyelinating Diseases

Unfortunately, CSF cytology and biochemistry of acute and chronic demyelinating diseases are not specific to certain diseases. CSF abnormalities usually reflect the inflammatory nature of the majority of the underlying disease processes. Nonetheless, CSF analysis plays an important role in the diagnosis and differential diagnosis when combined with anamnestic information, the clinical symptoms and course, and data from imaging studies.

5.4.1   Multiple Sclerosis

Cerebral spinal fluid from patients suffering from multiple sclerosis (MS) is characterized by mild lymphocytic pleocytosis. Cell counts rarely exceed 50/μl and may be within the normal range, i.e., < 5/μl. The presence of granulocytes should alert the cytologist to other potential diagnoses, e.g., Behçet's disease with CNS manifestations. Immunoglobulin-synthesizing B-lymphocytes are common (Fig. 5.4.1A). They are indicative of the underlying inflammatory process, and are rarely found in normal CSF. These cells show an excentric nucleus, and an increased cytoplasm/nuclear ratio compared with non-activated, resting lymphocytes (inset, see also Sect. 3.2). Storage of immunoglobulins is indicated by a more pronounced and basophilic cytoplasmic border (arrowheads). Even though immunoglobulins can also be shown by immunocytochemistry, this is usually not needed. Besides activated B-lymphocytes, mature plasma cells are also found in MS (Fig. 5.4.1B). They are characterized by more intense blue staining and are slightly larger than activated B-cells.

A hallmark of inflammatory CNS diseases, including MS, is the intrathecal synthesis of immunoglobulins, mostly IgG. This is reflected by a disproportionate increase in the CSF/serum ratio of IgG as seen in the quotient diagram (Fig. 5.4.1C) as well as the presence of oligoclonal IgG in CSF (Fig. 5.4.1D). These changes may be accompanied by a mild or less common moderate disturbance of the blood–CSF barrier (Fig. 5.4.1C). Again, a severe disturbance of the blood–CSF barrier (CSF/serum ratio of albumin $> 20 \times 10^{-3}$) should raise the possibility of a different diagnosis.

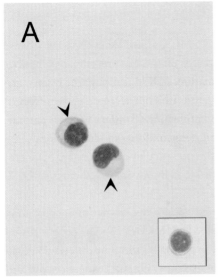

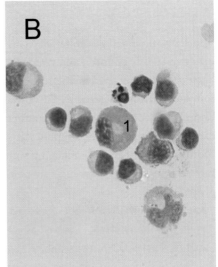

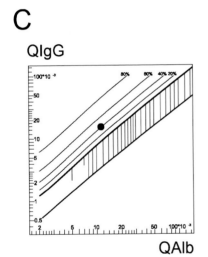

QIgG

QAlb

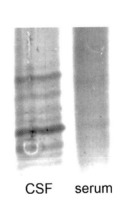

CSF   serum

5.4.2 Acute Disseminated Encephalomyelitis

Acute disseminated encephalomyelitis (ADEM) is a rare demyelinating disease affecting mostly children and young adults. It is oftentimes preceded by a viral or bacterial infection, e.g., measles, or a vaccination. ADEM is thought to be an autoimmune process triggered by the preceding infection or vaccination. Accordingly, CSF abnormalities are similar to other inflammatory disorders with an autoimmune pathogenesis, i.e., lymphocytic pleocytosis, mild to moderate blood–CSF barrier dysfunction, and less commonly the presence of oligoclonal IgG. Therefore, differentiation from an acute phase of MS is impossible on the basis of CSF analysis alone.

In CSF (Fig. 5.4.2A) one finds activated monocytes sometimes containing phagocytosed material (1) as well as activated lymphocytes (2). The phagocytosed material is derived from myelin sheaths. However, this cannot be differentiated on the basis of the routine cytology stains. A brain biopsy is usually not necessary and also not sufficient to make the diagnosis of ADEM. However, sometimes the possibility of other differential diagnoses requires a biopsy (Fig. 5.4.2B–D) demonstrating plenty of macrophages (Fig. 5.4.2B). By Luxol fast blue staining (Fig. 5.4.2C) the phagocytosed myelin sheaths lead to light blue staining of the cytoplasm of macrophages (1). Immunohistochemistry for neurofilament (Fig. 5.4.2D) often shows that the axons remain intact (brown reaction product) and are not attacked by phagocytic cells. One should keep in mind that the histology is nonspecific and compatible with demyelinating processes in general.

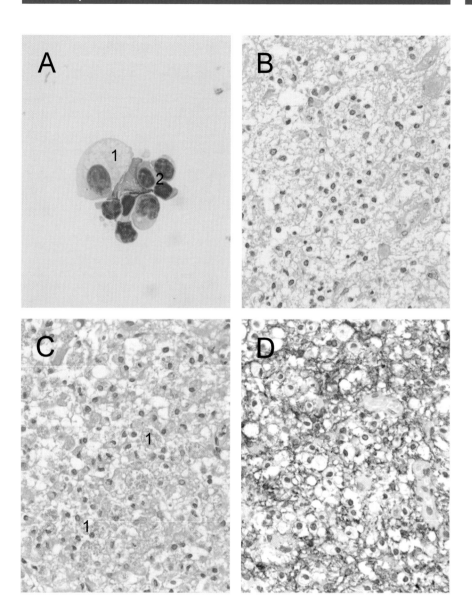

CHAPTER 6

Neoplastic Disorders

6.1 General Considerations

When microscopically examining slides from CSF specimens with suspected neoplastic meningitis, the investigator is typically confronted with one of the two principal constellations: either a primary malignancy is already known or at least suspected from radiological investigations, or clinical and neuroradiological findings are suggestive of neoplastic meningitis without sufficient evidence of the primary tumor. The latter situation is uncomfortable insofar as a non-neoplastic reactive process may sometimes closely mimic a neoplastic one in cytologic preparations. Furthermore, if undoubtedly malignant cells are detectable, it is frequently impossible to supply the clinician with precise details concerning location of the primary tumor or even information regarding the tumor entity. Admittedly, an experienced cytologist may achieve a high degree of diagnostic accuracy for some selected tumor entities – but if there are neuroradiologically distinguishable foci within the leptomeninges, a diagnostic leptomeningeal biopsy may help to definitely arrive at a reliable diagnosis. In the case of a known and ideally histopathologically diagnosed and classified primary tumor outside or inside the CNS, CSF cytology is typically carried out for staging purposes or for controlling therapy efforts. Then, the only question to be answered is: Are there any cells that are neoplastic or suspected of being neoplastic? Since meningeal seeding mostly occurs in patients with malignant primary tumors, it is indispensable to know the criteria for malignant cells, as there are:

- Abnormally large cells
- Large nuclei
- Increased polymorphism of nuclei
- Hyperchromatism of the nucleus
- Frequently inhomogeneous chromatin texture
- Increased number of nucleoli

- Nuclear fragments, looking like "accessory nuclei"
- Increased mitosis rate; however, one mitosis does not make a neoplasm and, vice versa, no or only few mitoses do not exclude a malignant tumor
- Pathological atypical mitoses
- Shift of the nuclear–cytoplasmic ratio
- Cytoplasm with intense blue color (basophilic) due to increased RNA content needed for enhanced protein synthesis
- Plurivacuolation as marker for an activated state due to increased metabolism
- Cytoplasmic bridges between neoplastic cells

If unequivocally malignant cells are present, a few such atypical cells are sufficient for the correct diagnosis of neoplastic meningitis. However, extreme caution is advisable when analyzing CSF slides from infants and young children where leptomeningeal cell clusters with a high proliferation rate may be present; these are harmless and no indicator of a neoplasm [9]. Furthermore, blast-like tumor cell clusters, thought to be of germinal matrix origin, are sometimes found in CSF of neonates and young infants, particularly in connection with a history of prematurity, hydrocephalus, or birth trauma, and must not be misinterpreted as neoplastic meningitis [10–12].

If there are only cells with suspected neoplasia, immunocytochemistry will be very helpful – provided that the neoplastic cells have maintained their expression characteristics. Unfortunately, however, the more malignant and dedifferentiated a tumor, the stronger the likelihood of loss of expression of specific marker proteins. Additional techniques, which in specific situations may substantially improve information regarding the classification "neoplastic or non-neoplastic," are immunophenotyping by flow cytometry, in situ hybridization [13], or the use of polymerase chain reaction. In the latter case, however, the genetic alteration of the primary neoplasia must be known. These techniques may be particularly valuable in diagnosing neoplastic cells in chronic forms of leukemia where differentiation from lymphocytic infiltration is extremely difficult and sometimes even impossible.

Another significant problem in practice is how to deal with a negative cytology, i.e., the absence of malignant cells or those with suspected neoplasia, despite strong clinical or neuroradiological evidence. While some authors claim that nearly every occurrence of neoplastic meningitis is detectable [9], it is reasonable to assume that, due to the multifocal nature of neoplastic meningitis, CSF obtained from sites distant from the pathological process may yield a negative cytology [14, 15]. Data from the literature suggest that up to 45% of cases will be cytologically negative at first examination, but up to 90% will be identified by means of a second CSF examination. Little benefit, however, will derive from additional repetitive punctures [16]. In general, malignant cells will appear in CSF most commonly when there is generalized seeding of the leptomeninges by tumor cells, less often when there is only focal seeding and almost never when the tumor is limited to the brain and the pial surface has not been breached [17]. If neuroradiologically suspect leptomeningeal or, in particular, intraparenchymal lesions are present, either a leptomeningeal or a stereotactic brain biopsy should be considered. Especially in the case of a suspected primary CNS lymphoma, with the patient's state of health being critical, no time should be wasted on repetitive punctures for CSF analysis, aiming at a diagnosis.

Since cytology deals with single cells, one difficulty in arriving at the correct diagnosis is lack of information concerning tumor architecture. Furthermore, due to environmental differences, tumor cells frequently show secondary changes in the CSF. Since, unfortunately, cytological diagnosis is frequently made by investigators unfamiliar with the histopathology of tumors, we have added some figures with typical histoarchitectural features, to give an impression of the primary tumor.

In summary, when neoplastic meningitis is suspected, the crucial question to be answered is: "Neoplastic cells/suspected neoplasia cells or not?" Knowledge consisting of clinical data, neuroradiologic findings, history, and location of the tumor is frequently essential to arrive at a correct diagnosis. Clusters of cells in CSF preparations from the ventricle may be confused with tumor cells when the investigator takes it for a CSF sample from a lumbar puncture.

6.2   Metastatic Tumors and Meningeal Carcinomatosis

6.2.1   Breast Cancer

Meningeal carcinomatosis occurs in up to 5% of patients with breast cancer [18]. Although small-cell lung cancer and melanoma have a higher percentage of leptomeningeal spread, breast cancer accounts for most cases due to its higher incidence [19]. There are two major types of breast carcinomas, tumors of ductal origin and tumors of lobular origin, which differ significantly in their cytologic presentation in CSF specimens. Tumors of ductal origin typically form large cell clusters (Fig. 6.2.1A, objective × 20). In the corresponding histology, a ductal invasive carcinoma of the breast has been diagnosed (Fig. 6.2.1B). In contrast to ductal tumors, lobular carcinomas (Fig. 6.2.1D) mostly have isolated tumor cells in CSF specimens. Characteristically, there are striking differences in size between single cells. However, this is not specific and may also be observed in CSF specimens with neoplastic cells from ductal breast carcinoma (Fig. 6.2.1C: an atypical mitosis is present, 1, objective × 20).

Useful antibodies
- Anti-pan-cytokeratin (MNF-116) or antibodies against specific cytokeratins to confirm the epithelial origin
- Anti-estrogen and/or progesterone receptor (if epithelial histogenesis has already been proven)

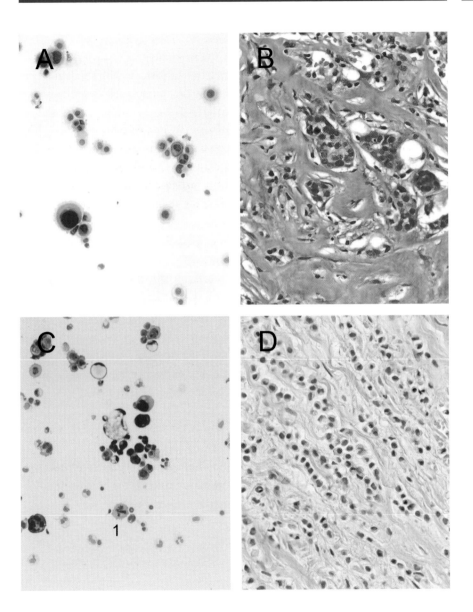

6.2.2   Lung Cancer

Compared with neoplastic meningitis in up to 6% of patients with small-cell lung cancer (SCLC), non-small-cell lung cancer (NSCLC) rarely causes meningeal carcinomatosis (approximately 1% incidence) [18]. If the neoplastic cells have retained their capacity to express marker proteins normally used for the classification of paraffin-embedded tissue, statements on tumor location or entity may be possible. As in the present case, adenocarcinomas mostly present as single cells (Fig. 6.2.2A, 1), but not as cell clusters. One or more prominent nucleoli are characteristic (Fig. 6.2.2A, arrowhead). In contrast to SCLC, a broad, strongly basophilic cytoplasm, with numerous vacuoles indicating a metabolically active state, is visible. Erythrocytes (Fig. 6.2.2A, 2), often present in CSF specimens, can be used for scale. Epithelial origin is demonstrated by strong immunostaining using an antibody against pan-cytokeratin (MNF-116; Fig. 6.2.2B). In this context, the use of an antibody against the thyroid transcription factor-1 (TTF-1) can be very helpful. If positive nuclear immunostaining as shown (Fig. 6.2.2C, arrowhead) can be demonstrated, location of the primary tumor in the lung or thyroid is most likely [20]. The corresponding tissue of the surgically resected lung tumor shows a moderately differentiated adenocarcinoma with cytoplasm-rich tumor cells (Fig. 6.2.2D), similar to those in the CSF specimen (Fig. 6.2.2A).

Useful antibodies
- Anti-pan-cytokeratin (MNF-116) or antibodies against specific cytokeratins
- Anti-TTF-1 (to confirm location of the primary tumor in the lung or thyroid)
- Anti-synaptophysin or other neuronal markers (as markers for SCLC)

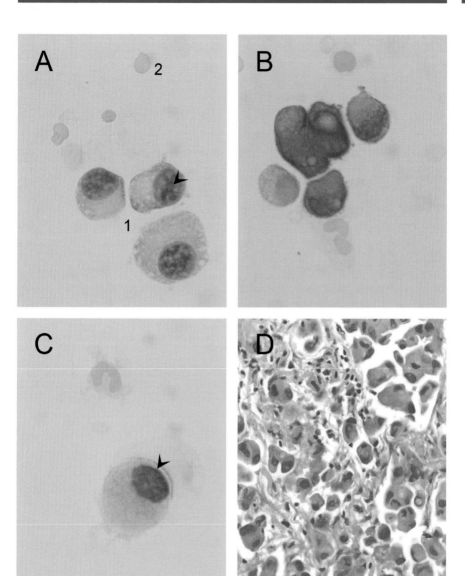

6.2.3   Gastric Cancer

Compared with carcinomas of the respiratory tract and breast, tumors of the gastrointestinal tract rarely lead to neoplastic meningitis (up to 0.25%) [18]. Some specific entities show rather characteristic features in cytologic specimens. In Fig. 6.2.3A, a cellular CSF specimen with densely packed atypical cells is shown. One cell (Fig. 6.2.3A, 1) shows the typical appearance of a signet ring with nuclei displaced to the border by mucous material in the center of the cell. Immunocytochemistry with an antibody against pan-cytokeratin (MNF-116) labels numerous cells and reveals multiple vacuoles within the cytoplasm (Fig. 6.2.3B, 1). In the paraffin-embedded material, the typical histological aspect of a signet cell carcinoma is present (Fig. 6.2.3C), exhibiting strongly PAS-positive material in the cytoplasm of the tumor cells (Fig. 6.2.3D).

Useful antibodies

- Anti-pan-cytokeratin (MNF-116) or antibodies against specific cytokeratins

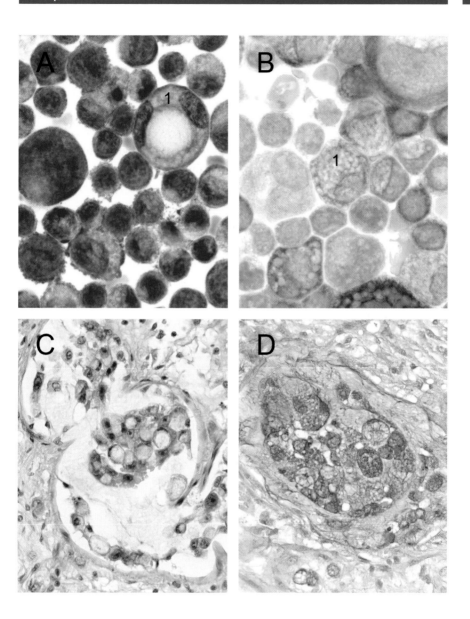

6.2.4   Malignant Melanoma

Epidemiological data on the incidence of leptomeningeal spread in patients with malignant melanoma differ markedly. Nevertheless, neoplastic meningitis, due to malignant melanoma, is not a rare event [18]. The cytologic preparations from CSF typically exhibit rather large tumor cells of varying size, with round nuclei and prominent nucleoli (Fig. 6.2.4A,B). The cytoplasm is sometimes frayed or shows bizarre protrusions (Fig. 6.2.4B, 1). If melanin pigment is present (Fig. 6.2.4B, 2), diagnosis can easily be made. In case of doubt, special stains for melanin (Fontana, Masson–Hampel) versus iron readily identify the nature of the pigment. Frequently, however, no melanin is detectable in neoplastic cells. Then, the first differential diagnosis based on cytological features is metastatic cancer. If clinical history is unavailable, immunocytochemical stains may be very helpful. A number of reliable antibodies for the detection of melanomas (HMB-45, anti-Melan A, anti-S-100) are available or, vice versa, immunostaining with a cytokeratin antibody (in our hands MNF-116 works excellently) may identify the epithelial origin. In Fig. 6.2.4C, two neoplastic cells are stained with an S-100 antibody, corroborating the suspected diagnosis of malignant melanoma. The typical histopathological aspect of malignant melanoma metastatic to the brain is shown in Fig. 6.2.4D with multiple cells stained by the HMB-45 antibody. If no primary tumor can be detected, the possibility of a primary melanotic lesion of the leptomeninges has to be considered [21]. Otherwise, regression of the primary tumor is a theoretical possibility [22].

Useful antibodies
- HMB-45 or anti-Melan A to confirm the melanotic nature
- Anti-S-100 as a helpful though unspecific marker
- Anti-pan-cytokeratin (MNF-116) to potentially identify an epithelial primary

Figure 6.2.4A was kindly provided by Professor Bergmann, Bremen, Germany; Fig. 6.2.4B was kindly provided by Professor Birklein, Mainz, Germany.

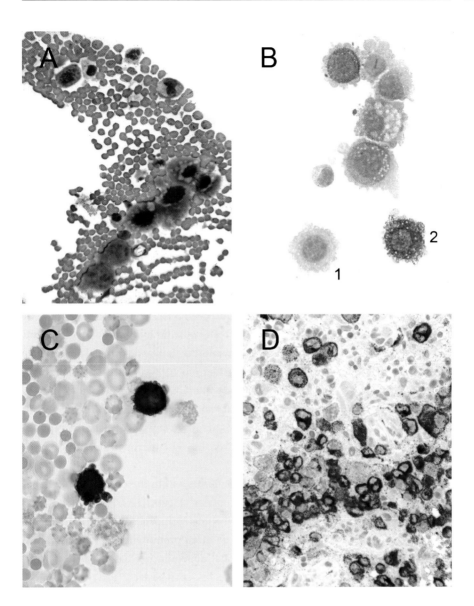

6.3 Hematologic Neoplasms

6.3.1 Leukemia

Neoplastic meningitis is rarely the initial presentation in patients with leukemia or lymphoma. The typical situation is a CSF examination for staging or treatment control. According to the conventional FAB (French–American–British) classification, leukemia can be classified as acute and chronic types, and further subclassified as lymphoid and myeloid types. Although accepted for many years, the discovery of a number of genetic lesions that predict clinical behavior and outcome better than morphology and other molecular genetic data forced a new classification scheme. According to the current WHO classification [23], four major groups of myeloid diseases can be distinguished: chronic myeloproliferative diseases, myelodysplastic/myeloproliferative diseases, myelodysplastic syndromes, and acute myeloid leukemia. The exact classification is based on a combination of morphology, immunophenotype, and cytogenetic features from blood and bone marrow. When analyzing CSF cytology, subclassification of leukemia has usually already been performed, and the only remaining issue to be determined is whether or not neoplastic meningitis is present. Acute leukemia, in particular acute lymphoblastic leukemia (ALL), carries the highest risk of leptomeningeal spread. While acute myeloid leukemia (AML) only infrequently causes neoplastic meningitis, one subtype, acute myelomonocytic leukemia, has a high propensity to invade the leptomeninges [24].

The typical cytologic aspects of leukemic blasts within the CSF are varying size and only scant or completely invisible cytoplasm (Fig. 6.3.1A). Nuclei are irregular and convoluted, with finely dispersed chromatin and, according to the lineage and grade of maturation, with none, one or more prominent nucleoli (as shown in Fig. 6.3.1A), resulting in the typical "blast" appearance. Characteristically, isolated single tumor cells rather than clustered cells can be seen (Fig. 6.3.1B). However, due to a high cell count, this phenomenon may be masked (Fig. 6.3.1A). In Fig. 6.3.1C and D some further characteristics of acute leukemia cells are shown. Nuclear protrusions (Fig. 6.3.1C, arrowhead), as seen in this CSF from a patient with ALL, are a typical finding. Nuclear fragments looking like "accessory nuclei" are unspecific criteria in malignant cells and often present in neoplastic cells in hematological disorders (Fig. 6.3.1D, arrowhead). False-positive CSF findings may derive from contamination of the specimen by fresh blood, lacking the phenomenon of erythrophagia or detectable hemosiderin. Knowledge of the peripheral blood count is essential. In chronic forms, the cytological criteria for malignancy may be less pronounced. Detailed information concerning the subtype should be provided by the physician to facilitate correct diagnosis. CLL or CML combined with pleocytosis is either due to additional inflammation or, if blasts can unequivocally be identified, transformation into a high-grade neoplasm must be assumed.

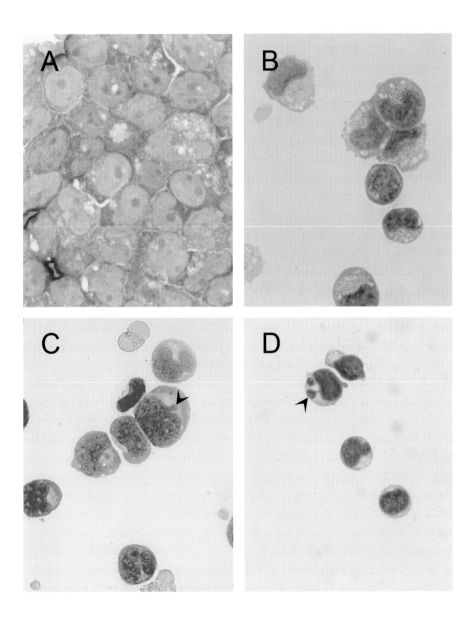

6.3.2   Lymphoma

According to the current WHO classification [23], lymphomas are classified as B-cell neoplasms, T- and NK cell neoplasms, or Hodgkin's lymphoma. Within the category of "non-Hodgkin's" lymphoma (NHL), a large number of distinct diseases associated with distinctive epidemiology, etiology, clinical features, and, often, distinctive responses to therapy are included. While Hodgkin's lymphoma very rarely involves the leptomeninges, neoplastic meningitis commonly occurs in NHL patients. Primary CNS lymphoma, which in approximately 90% of cases belongs to the group of diffuse large B-cell lymphomas, results in a positive cytology from initial CSF specimens in only up to 15% of patients [25]. Therefore, patients with progressive clinical symptoms should immediately undergo stereotactic brain biopsy for fast and definitive diagnosis [26]. Similar to acute leukemia, neoplastic cells of high-grade lymphomas in CSF specimens can readily be identified by their blast-like appearance. The differentiation between B- and T-cell lymphoma is usually not an issue for the interpretation of CSF specimens, since the exact lymphoma subtype has most often already been determined based on other tissues. Normally, the investigator faces the pivotal question of: "Neoplastic meningitis, yes or no?" In principle, however, subclassification is also possible by means of immunocytochemistry.

Figure 6.3.2A shows a typical example of delayed CSF submission to the investigating laboratory, resulting in a cytologic preparation containing only vaguely recognizable, but highly suspect, atypical large cells (Fig. 6.3.2A, 1). A correctly performed cytologic CSF examination from the same patient (Fig. 6.3.2B) shows large atypical cells with conspicuously convoluted nuclei, prominent nucleoli and basophilic cytoplasm (Fig. 6.3.2B, 1), demonstrating lymphomatous meningitis of the clinically known high-grade NHL. Due to cytostatic therapy with methotrexate, one neoplastic cell is undergoing apoptosis (Fig. 6.3.2B, 2). A classic diagnostic pitfall is seen in Fig. 6.3.2C (objective × 20) and at higher magnification in Fig. 6.3.2D (oil immersion, objective × 100). Diagnosis of neoplastic meningitis, due to the cerebrospinal spread of a low-grade lymphoma, is difficult, since the cells do not show any atypical features. However, additional flow cytometric analysis clearly demonstrated the neoplastic nature of these cells. Similar to chronic leukemia, low-grade NHL combined with pleocytosis is either due to additional inflammation or, when blasts are unequivocally identified, transformation into a high-grade neoplasm must be assumed. One major pitfall is the differentiation between reactive pleocytosis with blast-like elements and neoplastic meningitis. A helpful feature in this context is that various stages of activation are typically detectable in infectious lesions mimicking neoplastic meningitis.

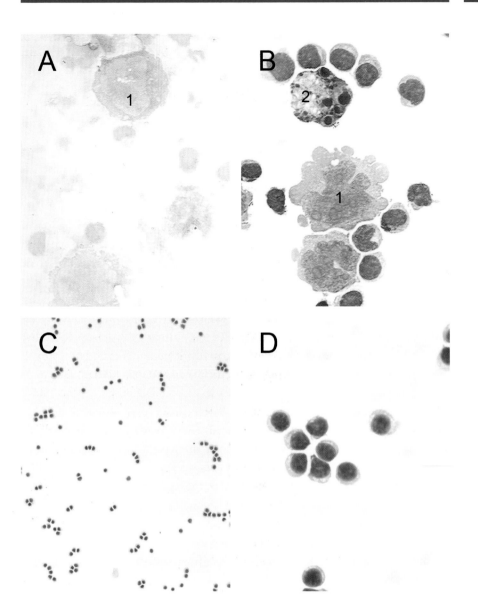

6.4 Primary Central Nervous System Neoplasms

6.4.1   Astrocytic Tumors

6.4.1.1 *Anaplastic Astrocytoma*

While, in principle, all astrocytic tumors and, in particular, the anaplastic vari-
ants, have the potential for leptomeningeal spread and dissemination via the cerebrospinal pathways, CSF samples for primary cytologic diagnosis are of very
limited value. Unfortunately, in the rare cases of primary leptomeningeal gliomas,
where diagnosis from cytologic specimens would be helpful, detection of tumor
cells in CSF samples is a rare exception [27]. Similarly, reports on spinal low-grade
gliomas with extensive leptomeningeal dissemination indicate that CSF findings
are largely restricted to elevated protein, while neoplastic cells are not detectable
[28]. Furthermore, while pilocytic astrocytomas (WHO grade I) frequently in-
filtrate the leptomeningeal space (Fig. 6.4.1.1A, 1) histologic specimen, objective
×5), true dissemination via the CSF is largely restricted to pilocytic astrocytomas
of the hypothalamic/chiasmatic region in infants and young children. Due to its
characteristic morphological features and a less favourable prognosis this tumor
has been listed as a variant in the current WHO classification, the so-called pilomyxoid astrocytoma (WHO grade II) [29, 30]. The classic situation in which the
neuropathologist faces the pivotal question of presence or absence of neoplastic
astrocytic cells in CSF samples, concerns either a known astrocytic tumor or a
check for tumor cells in the CSF for control purposes.

Morphology of astrocytic tumor cells in CSF samples is variable and fulfills the
general criteria for malignant cells. Figure 6.4.1.1B is a typical example of rather
large cells with broad, sometimes vacuolated cytoplasm (Fig. 6.4.1.1B, 1). Nuclei
are mildly pleomorphic, hyperchromatic, and possess distinct nucleoli. The corresponding histologic specimens (Fig. 6.4.1.1C, D) show an astrocytic tumor that
has developed multiple subependymal protrusions from which dissemination into
the ventricular CSF is easy to imagine. Glial histogenesis is confirmed by glial
fibrillary acidic protein (GFAP) immunohistochemistry (Fig. 6.4.1.1D). Due to its
cell pleomorphism and increased proliferation index, this tumor has been classified as an anaplastic astrocytoma (WHO grade III).

Useful antibodies

- Anti-GFAP (to clarify glial histogenesis of tumor cells, although GFAP immunoreactivity does not automatically indicate a neoplastic or astrocytic cell; anaplastic glial cells, however, not infrequently lose their GFAP expression)
- Anti-MAP2 (normally expressed in neuronal cells, MAP2 can also be used as a marker for glial histogenesis of tumor cells/progenitors)

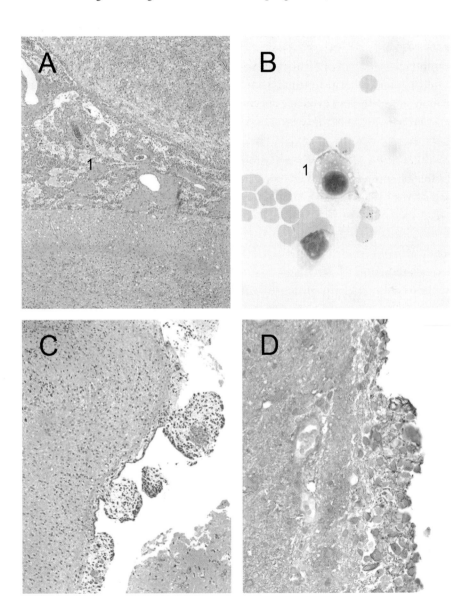

6.4.1.2 *Glioblastoma Multiforme*

Glioblastoma multiforme (GBM) is the most common and most malignant glioma (WHO grade IV) in adults. Despite its highly infiltrative growth manner, metastasis via cerebrospinal pathways is rather rare. GBM may show the highest degree of anaplasia and pleomorphism. In Fig. 6.4.1.2A, a highly anaplastic cell (1) can be seen with a hyperchromatic nucleus containing numerous nucleoli. Furthermore, multiple bizarre cytoplasmic protrusions are detectable. In addition, some activated lymphocytes (2), monocytes (3), and erythrocytes (4) can be seen. In Fig. 6.4.1.2B, a neoplastic cell with prominent nucleoli and basophilic, plurivacuolated cytoplasm is present (1). Apart from GFAP immunostaining, immunohistochemistry with an antibody against the microtubule-associated protein-2 (MAP2) may be a useful tool for the detection of neoplastic glial cells (Fig. 6.4.1.2C, 1). Although primarily regarded as a neuronal marker protein, MAP2 is now a recognized marker for glial progenitors [31]. The corresponding histologic specimen shows an anaplastic tumor of high cell density with palisading necrosis (Fig. 6.4.1.2D, 1), fulfilling all histological criteria for a diagnosis of GBM.

6

Useful antibodies

- Anti-GFAP (to clarify glial histogenesis of tumor cells, although GFAP immunoreactivity does not automatically indicate a neoplastic or astrocytic cell)
- Anti-MAP2 (normally expressed in neuronal cells, MAP2 can also be used as a marker for glial histogenesis of tumor cells/progenitors)

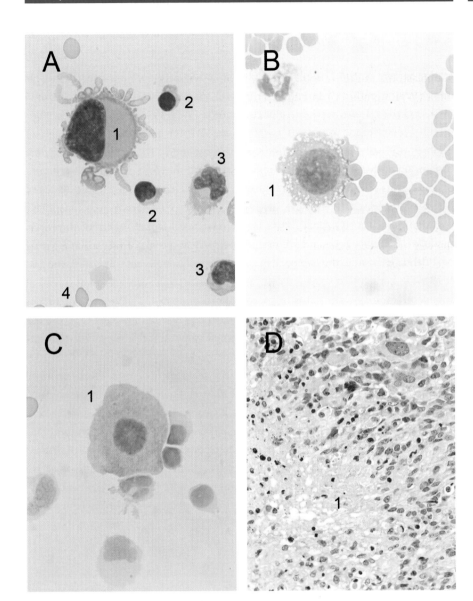

6.4.2   Ependymal Tumors

In the current WHO classification [30], ependymal tumors are subclassified as the following entities: ependymoma (WHO grade II), anaplastic ependymoma (WHO grade III), myxopapillary ependymoma (WHO grade I), and subependymoma (WHO grade I). Ependymoblastomas (WHO grade IV), rare malignant brain tumors affecting young children, are assigned to the group of embryonal tumors. Ependymomas arise throughout the CNS in close proximity to the ependyma or its remnants. Most commonly, they develop in the posterior fossa and the spinal cord where they are the most common glial tumors. Myxopapillary ependymomas (WHO grade I) are largely restricted to the region of the conus medullaris, cauda equina and filum terminale of the spinal cord. Surrounded only by a delicate capsule, the tumor may spontaneously penetrate this soft tissue and seed the subarachnoid space. In contrast, reference to the cerebrospinal spread of subependymomas is restricted to anecdotal case reports [32]. While up to 15% of patients with ependymomas have disseminated disease at diagnosis [33], the use of CSF analysis for disease staging is of limited value, since the negativity of lumbar CSF samples is of low predictive significance [34].

Ependymal cells show some characteristic features. In contrast to, astrocytic cells, for example, nuclei are mostly somewhat elongated, relatively isomorphic, and show distinct micronucleoli (Fig. 6.4.2A, objective ×40; B, oil immersion). Sometimes, fine processes are detectable. Cells from differentiated ependymomas may sometimes exhibit a macrophage-like appearance. Frequently, ependymal tumor cells are built up into cohesive cell conglomerates (Fig. 6.4.2C, objective ×20). The corresponding histologic specimen shows a mucinous dissociated tumor with monomorphic cells and broad fibrotic tissue typical of myxopapillary ependymoma (Fig. 6.4.2D).

Useful antibodies
- Anti-GFAP (typically, ependymoma cells demonstrate strong GFAP immunostaining; however, as already stated for astrocytomas, GFAP immunoreactivity does not automatically indicate a neoplastic or ependymal cell)

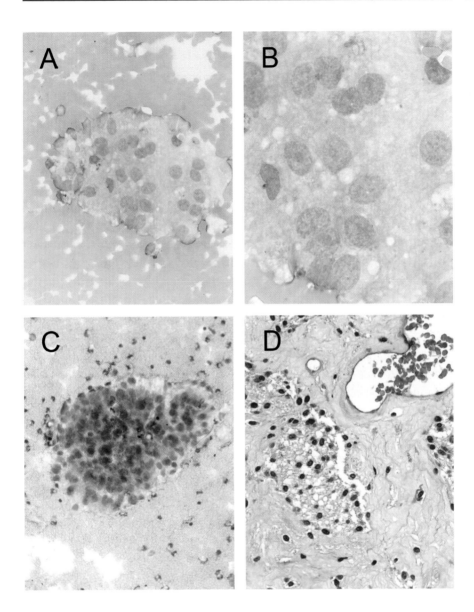

6.4.3   Embryonal Tumors/Central Nervous System Primitive Neuroectodermal Tumors (WHO Grade IV)

6.4.3.1 *Medulloblastoma*

The medulloblastoma is the most common example of the group of embryonal tumors occurring in the brain. As already stated in the WHO definition of this tumor [30], medulloblastomas show an "inherent tendency to metastasize via CSF pathways." Due to this behavior, approximately one-third of patients present with metastasis at diagnosis. Primary diagnosis from CSF samples is rare, since patients with medulloblastomas usually present with high intracranial pressure, in which case lumbar puncture is forbidden. In cytologic preparations from CSF samples, medulloblastoma cells typically occur in cell clusters (Fig. 6.4.3.1/6.4.3.2A). The neoplastic cells mostly possess small, plump nuclei ranging from round (1) to oval (2) or turnip-shaped (3). Typically, there is a shift in the nuclear-to-cytoplasmic ratio with only scant cytoplasm (Fig. 6.4.3.1/6.4.3.2A). As differential diagnoses, other embryonal tumors or a small-cell carcinoma of the lung have to be considered. However, clinical data and location of the primary tumor are helpful in arriving at the correct diagnosis. The corresponding paraffin-embedded material shows a highly cellular embryonal tumor (Fig. 6.4.3.1/6.4.3.2B) with a tendency to form primitive neuroblastic rosettes (arrowheads).

6.4.3.2 *Retinoblastoma*

The retinoblastoma (which is not listed in the current WHO classification of tumors of the central nervous system) is a retinal embryonal neoplasm that either extends directly from an ocular lesion or presents as a primary intracerebral lesion in the pineal or suprasellar region as part of the "trilateral retinoblastoma" complex. Advanced tumors may break through the optic nerve and enter the subarachnoid space. The cytological preparation shows neoplastic cells that are mostly indistinguishable from other embryonal neoplasms (Fig. 6.4.3.1/6.4.3.2C; cf. A). The same holds true for the histologic specimens. Again, a highly cellular embryonal tumor is present (Fig. 6.4.3.1/6.4.3.2D; cf. B). Incidentally, scattered apoptotic cells are visible (Fig. 6.4.3.1/6.4.3.2D, arrowheads). If distinctive features, such as Flexner–Wintersteiner rosettes or "fleurettes" are lacking (Fig. 6.4.3.1/6.4.3.2D), diagnosis cannot be made without additional clinical information or special immunohistochemical stains.

Useful antibodies

- Anti-synaptophysin or other neuronal marker proteins may be helpful if the tumor shows a tendency toward neuronal differentiation. In the context of clinical data, however, immunocytochemistry is seldom necessary, due to the characteristic cytology of the tumor cells

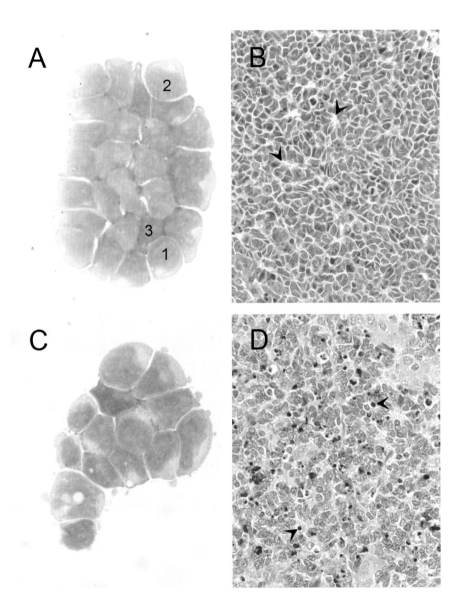

6.4.3.3 *Atypical Teratoid/Rhabdoid Tumor*

Like CNS-primitive neuroectodermal tumors, the atypical teratoid/rhabdoid tumor (AT/RT) belongs to the group of embryonal tumors corresponding to WHO grade IV (malignant). The great majority of AT/RTs manifest in children, usually less than 2 years old. About half of AT/RTs arise in the posterior fossa, followed in frequency of occurrence by supratentorial locations. At presentation, about 30% of patients already have manifest dissemination via CSF pathways. CSF specimens show isolated (Fig. 6.4.3.3A) or clustered (Fig. 6.4.3.3B) tumor cells with abundant cytoplasm and chromatin-dense nuclei. Mitoses (Fig. 6.4.3.3B, 1) are frequently seen, although, as a general principle in CSF diagnosis, the absence of mitoses does not exclude malignancy. The typical rhabdoid aspect is maintained in the cytologic specimen (Fig. 6.4.3.3A,B), compared with the corresponding histology from paraffin-embedded material (Fig. 6.4.3.3C,D). Rhabdoid cells may contain an inclusion-like pink structure (Fig. 6.4.3.3C, arrowhead), which is even more clearly visible in the cytologic preparation (Fig. 6.4.3.3A, arrowheads; B, arrowhead). Strong vimentin immunoreactivity, though not specific, is characteristically seen in rhabdoid cells of AT/RTs (Fig. 6.4.3.3D). The penetration of tumor cells through the ependymal layer and invasion of the ventricular system are convincingly demonstrated (Fig. 6.4.3.3D). The rate of rhabdoid cells may vary and is usually accompanied by primitive neuroectodermal, mesenchymal, and epithelial cells (not shown).

Useful antibodies
- Anti-vimentin (however, specificity is very low)

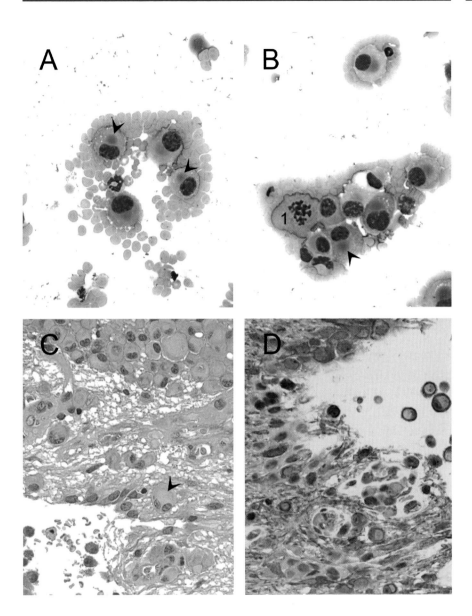

6.4.4   Germ Cell Tumors; Germinoma

Most CNS germ cell tumors develop in the midline structures of children and adolescents with the pinealis region as the most common site of origin, followed by the suprasellar region. Intracerebral germ cell tumors, however, may also be metastases arising from the gonads. Like their extracranial counterparts, intracranial germ cell tumors can be divided into germinomas and non-germinomatous tumors, which can be further sub-classified as embryonal carcinoma, choriocarcinoma, yolk sac tumor, and teratoma. Mixed germ cell tumors also occur. Since prognosis and therapy differ significantly if additional non-germinomatous components are present, careful examination is indispensable for an exact diagnosis. Analysis of the pattern of marker proteins in the CSF (AFP, CEA, beta-HCG, PLAP) may be helpful in indicating the components present. Germ cell tumors have a high tendency to disseminate via CSF pathways. While CSF cytological analysis is well established for staging and control investigations, primary diagnosis of intracranial germ cell tumors is the domain of stereotactic brain biopsy.

Central nervous system germinomas are histologically identical to gonadal seminomas and dysgerminomas of the ovary. Cytological preparations from pure germinomas typically reveal large, mostly polygonal tumor cells with large vesicular nuclei and prominent nucleoli (Fig. 6.4.4.1A, 1). As in the histologic specimen (Fig. 6.4.4.1C), a strikingly reactive lymphocytic component is frequently present (Fig. 6.4.4.1A, 2; B, 1). Sometimes, even more pleomorphic cells are detectable (Fig. 6.4.4.1B, 2). Very similar cytologic features are seen in the corresponding histology. Again, large cells with abundant cytoplasm and vesicular nucleoli are visible (Fig. 6.4.4.1C, 1). Immunohistochemistry against placental alkaline phosphatase (PLAP) confirms the diagnosis of a germinoma (Fig. 6.4.4.1, D) and may also be of diagnostic use in cytologic specimens. Recently, OCT4 (also called OCT3, OTF3, POU5F1), a 18-kDa POU-domain transcription factor, has been shown to serve as a specific marker for CNS germinoma that is superior to the usual PLAP immunohistochemistry [35–37].

Useful antibodies
- Anti-PLAP
- Anti-OCT4

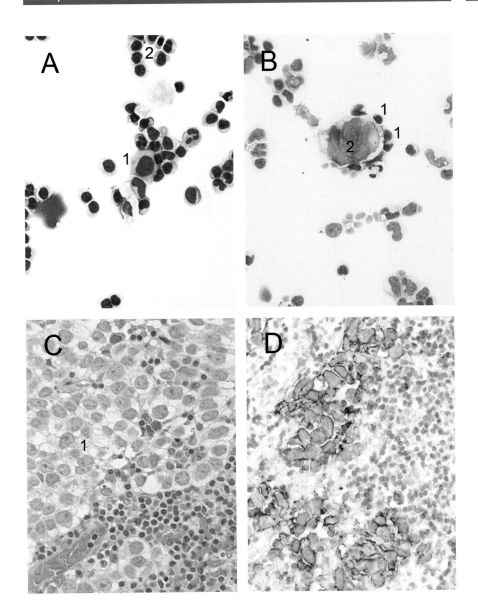

6.4.5   Choroid Plexus Tumors

While choroid plexus carcinomas (WHO grade III) frequently metastasize via cerebrospinal pathways, this is a rare event in choroid plexus papillomas (WHO grade I) [38]. Morphologically, normal choroid plexus cells (Fig. 6.4.5A: histologic specimen) are indistinguishable from cells derived from a differentiated choroid plexus papilloma (Fig. 6.4.5B: histologic specimen, objective × 10). This may pose a diagnostic problem, particularly in CSF specimens from the ventricle, where small pieces of normal choroid plexus are not infrequently present (see Sect. 3.5). Single cells from a choroid plexus carcinoma, which is readily identified in the histologic specimen (Fig. 6.4.5C), may also be cytologically indistinguishable from normal choroid plexus or choroid plexus papilloma. Origin in the choroid plexus can be demonstrated by use of some newly described antibodies against an inward rectifier potassium channel Kir7.1 (Fig. 6.4.5D) or the glycoprotein stanniocalcin-1, which seems to be highly specific for plexus tissue [39]. This may be particularly helpful, if a differential diagnosis of metastatic carcinoma versus malignant dedifferentiated plexus tumor arises.

Useful antibodies

- Anti-Kir7.1 (seems to be very specific for plexus epithelium, both normal and neoplastic)

Figure 6.4.5D was kindly provided by Professor Paulus, Münster, Germany.

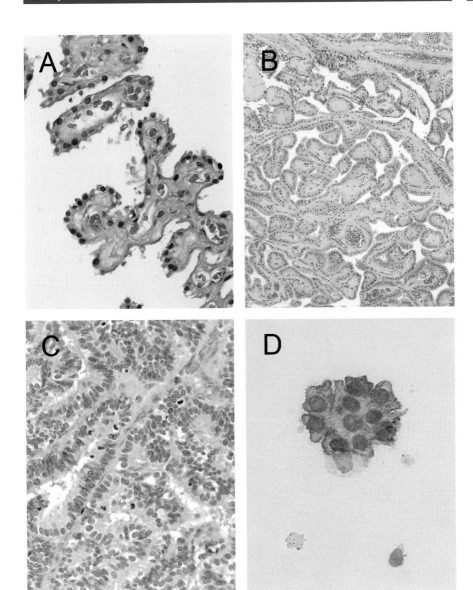

CHAPTER 7   Contaminants

7.1 General Considerations

Contamination of cytospin preparations with foreign elements is a common phenomenon. These foreign elements may be of various sizes and of either living (e.g., bacteria, fungi, pollen) or non-living (e.g., starch) origin. In the majority of cases, contamination can be avoided by education of both the clinical and laboratory staff and by altered management of CSF. In general, it is helpful to pay attention to concomitant cells. If contamination does occur, the lack of inflammatory cells reveals these particles to be the contaminants.

7.2 Bacterial and Fungal Contamination

Procedural error in carrying out lumbar puncture, contamination of cytocentri-fuge funnels or automated Gram-staining apparatus results in pseudomeningitis, i.e., false-positive occurrence of bacteria (Fig. 7.2A,B) and/or fungi (Fig. 7.2C,D, objective ×20) in cytocentrifuge preparations. *Staphylococcus epidermidis* is said to be the most common contaminant. Bacterial and/or fungal contamina-tion may cause confusion, in particular if bacteria concur with monocytic cell forms, suggesting cellular uptake (Fig. 7.2B, arrowhead). However, mixed growth (Fig. 7.2A,B), as well as lack of increased numbers of inflammatory cells in a sam-ple of CSF (Fig. 7.2A–D), particularly a component of polymorphonuclear leuko-cytes or enlarged and atypical lymphocytes, suggests that pseudomeningitis rather than an infectious process may be present. In addition, the cell counts and glucose and lactate concentrations in the CSF may also be helpful in this case.

7

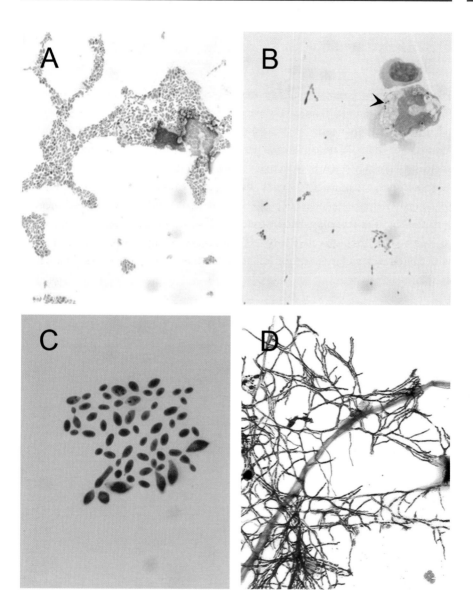

7.3 Pollen and Starch

When interpreting smears and specimens one can be misled by particles mimicking micro-organisms, especially parasites such as protozoa, mycotic agents or helminths. Although some of these pitfalls are well-known, others can be problematic. For example, false protozoa parasites can correspond to exogenous agents such as pollen (Fig. 7.3A,B, objective × 40).

Sometimes, the powder of gloves (starch) contaminating the specimen may be misinterpreted as cryptococci (Fig. 7.3C, objective × 40). However, in this case polarized light microscopy demonstrates the characteristic Maltese cross imaging of starch (Fig. 7.3D, objective × 40). Furthermore, in the case of contamination with pollen or starch the lack of inflammatory cells reveals these particles to be contaminants.

7

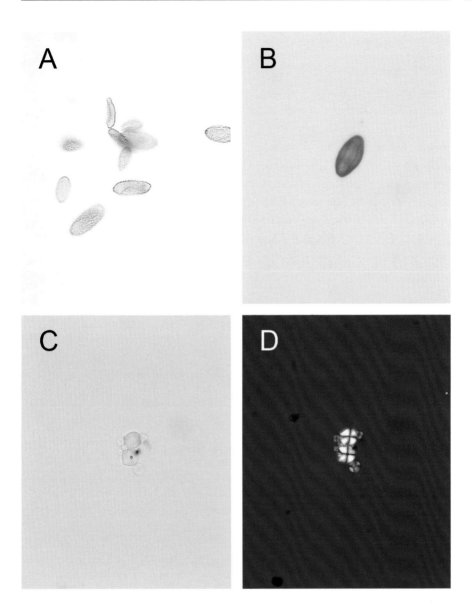

References

1. Kluge H, Wieczorek V, Linke E, Zimmermann K, Isenmann S, Witte OW (2007) Atlas of CSF cytology, 1st edn. Thieme, Stuttgart
2. Cserr HF (1971) Physiology of the choroid plexus. Physiol Rev 51:273–311
3. Kolar O, Zeman W (1968) Spinal fluid cytomorphology. Description of apparatus, technique, findings. Arch Neurol 18:44–51
4. Sornas R (1972) The cytology of the normal cerebrospinal fluid. Acta Neurol Scand 48:313–320
5. Svenningson A, Anderson O, Edsbagge M, et al. (1995) Lymphocyte phenotype and subset distribution in normal cerebrospinal fluid. J Neuroimmunol 63:39–46
6. Oehmichen M, Domasch D, Wietholter H (1982) Origin, proliferation, and fate of cerebrospinal fluid cells. A review on cerebrospinal fluid cell kinetics. J Neurol 227:145–150
7. Engelhardt P (1975) Diagnostic value of siderophages in the cytogram of cerebrospinal fluid. J Neurol 208:201–206
8. Petry F, Torzewski M, Bohl J, et al. (2006) Early diagnosis of Acanthamoeba infection during routine cytological examination of cerebrospinal fluid. J Clin Microbiol 44:1903–1904
9. Kolmel HW (1998) Cytology of neoplastic meningosis. J Neurooncol 38:121–125
10. Fernandes SP, Penchansky L (1996) Tumorlike clusters of immature cells in cerebrospinal fluid of infants. Pediatr Pathol Lab Med 16:721–729
11. Fischer JR, Davey DD, Gulley ML, et al. (1989) Blast-like cells in cerebrospinal fluid of neonates. Possible germinal matrix origin. Am J Clin Pathol 91:255–258
12. Jaffey PB, Varma SK, DeMay RM, et al. (1996) Blast-like cells in the cerebrospinal fluid of young infants: further characterization of clinical setting, morphology and origin. Am J Clin Pathol 105:544–547
13. Van Oostenbrugge RJ, Hopman AH, Ramaekers FC, et al. (1998) In situ hybridization: a possible diagnostic aid in leptomeningeal metastasis. J Neurooncol 38:127–133
14. Murray JJ, Greco FA, Wolff SN, et al. (1983) Neoplastic meningitis. Marked variations of cerebrospinal fluid composition in the absence of extradural block. Am J Med 75:289–294
15. Rogers LR, Duchesneau PM, Nunez C, et al. (1992) Comparison of cisternal and lumbar CSF examination in leptomeningeal metastasis. Neurology 42:1239–1241
16. Wasserstrom WR, Glass JP, Posner JB (1982) Diagnosis and treatment of leptomeningeal metastases from solid tumors: experience with 90 patients. Cancer 49:759–772

17. Glass JP, Melamed M, Chernik NL, et al. (1979) Malignant cells in cerebrospinal fluid (CSF): the meaning of a positive CSF cytology. Neurology 29:1369–1375

18. Gleissner B, Chamberlain MC (2006) Neoplastic meningitis. Lancet Neurol 5:443–452

19. Chamberlain MC (2005) Neoplastic meningitis. J Clin Oncol 23:3605–3613

20. Srodon M, Westra WH (2002) Immunohistochemical staining for thyroid transcription factor-1: a helpful aid in discerning primary site of tumor origin in patients with brain metastases. Hum Pathol 33:642–645

21. Brat DJ, Giannini C, Scheithauer BW, et al. (1999) Primary melanocytic neoplasms of the central nervous systems. Am J Surg Pathol 23:745–754

22. Katz KA, Jonasch E, Hodi FS, et al. (2005) Melanoma of unknown primary: experience at Massachusetts General Hospital and Dana-Farber Cancer Institute. Melanoma Res 15:77–82

23. Jaffe ES, Harris NL, Stein H, Vardiman JW (eds) (2001) WHO classification of tumours. Pathology and genetics of tumours of haematopoietic and lymphoid tissues, 2nd edn. IARC, Lyon

24. Chamberlain MC, Nolan C, Abrey LE (2005) Leukemic and lymphomatous meningitis: incidence, prognosis and treatment. J Neurooncol 75:71–83

25. Balmaceda C, Gaynor JJ, Sun M, et al. (1995) Leptomeningeal tumor in primary central nervous system lymphoma: recognition, significance, and implications. Ann Neurol 38:202–209

26. Batchelor T, Loeffler JS (2006) Primary CNS lymphoma. J Clin Oncol 24:1281–1288

27. Riva M, Bacigaluppi S, Galli C, et al. (2005) Primary leptomeningeal gliomatosis: case report and review of the literature. Neurol Sci 26:129–134

28. Perilongo G, Gardiman M, Bisaglia L, et al. (2002) Spinal low-grade neoplasms with extensive leptomeningeal dissemination in children. Childs Nerv Syst 18:505–512

29. Tihan T, Fisher PG, Kepner JL, et al. (1999) Pediatric astrocytomas with monomorphous pilomyxoid features and a less favorable outcome. J Neuropathol Exp Neurol 58:1061–1068

30. Louis DN, Ohgaki H, Wiestler OD, Cavenee WK (eds) (2007) WHO classification of tumours of the central nervous system, 4th edn. IARC, Lyon

31. Blümcke I, Muller S, Buslei R, et al. (2004) Microtubule-associated protein-2 immunoreactivity: a useful tool in the differential diagnosis of low-grade neuroepithelial tumors. Acta Neuropathol (Berl) 108:89–96

32. Seol HJ, Hwang SK, Choi YL, et al. (2003) A case of recurrent subependymoma with subependymal seeding: case report. J Neurooncol 62:315–320

33. Lassaletta A, Perez-Olleros P, Scaglione C, et al. (2007) Successful treatment of intracranial ependymoma with leptomeningeal spread with systemic chemotherapy and intrathecal liposomal cytarabine in a two-year-old child. J Neurooncol 24:24

34. Merchant TE, Fouladi M (2005) Ependymoma: new therapeutic approaches including radiation and chemotherapy. J Neurooncol 75:287–299

35. Hattab EM, Tu PH, Wilson JD, et al. (2005) OCT4 immunohistochemistry is superior to placental alkaline phosphatase (PLAP) in the diagnosis of central nervous system germinoma. Am J Surg Pathol 29:368–371

36. Cheng L, Sung MT, Cossu-Rocca P, et al. (2007) OCT4: biological functions and clinical applications as a marker of germ cell neoplasia. J Pathol 211:1–9
37. Takei H, Bhattacharjee MB, Rivera A, et al. (2007) New immunohistochemical markers in the evaluation of central nervous system tumors: a review of 7 selected adult and pediatric brain tumors. Arch Pathol Lab Med 131:234–241
38. McEvoy AW, Galloway M, Revesz T, et al. (2002) Metastatic choroid plexus papilloma: a case report. J Neurooncol 56:241–246
39. Hasselblatt M, Bohm C, Tatenhorst L, et al. (2006) Identification of novel diagnostic markers for choroid plexus tumors: a microarray-based approach. Am J Surg Pathol 30:66–74

Subject Index

Printing: Krips bv, Meppel, The Netherlands
Binding: Stürtz, Würzburg, Germany